Maurice J. Elias, Ph.
Joseph E. Zins, EdD
Editors

Bullying, Peer Harassment and Victimization in the Schools: The Next Generation of Prevention

Bullying, Peer Harassment and Victimization in the Schools: The Next Generation of Prevention has been co-published simultaneously as *Journal of Applied School Psychology*, Volume 19, Number 2 2003.

Pre-publication
REVIEWS,
COMMENTARIES,
EVALUATIONS . . .

The Haworth Press, Inc.

Bullying, Peer Harassment, and Victimization in the Schools: The Next Generation of Prevention

Bullying, Peer Harassment, and Victimization in the Schools: The Next Generation of Prevention has been co-published simultaneously as *Journal of Applied School Psychology*, Volume 19, Number 2 2003.

The *Journal of Applied School Psychology* Monographic "Separates"

Below is a list of "separates," which in serials librarianship means a special issue simultaneously published as a special journal issue or double-issue *and* as a "separate" hardbound monograph. (This is a format which we also call a "DocuSerial.")

"Separates" are published because specialized libraries or professionals may wish to purchase a specific thematic issue by itself in a format which can be separately cataloged and shelved, as opposed to purchasing the journal on an on-going basis. Faculty members may also more easily consider a "separate" for classroom adoption.

"Separates" are carefully classified separately with the major book jobbers so that the journal tie-in can be noted on new book order slips to avoid duplicate purchasing.

You may wish to visit Haworth's website at . . .

http://www.HaworthPress.com

. . . to search our online catalog for complete tables of contents of these separates and related publications.

You may also call 1-800-HAWORTH (outside US/Canada: 607-722-5857), or Fax 1-800-895-0582 (outside US/Canada: 607-771-0012), or e-mail at:

docdelivery@haworthpress.com

Bullying, Peer Harassment, and Victimization in the Schools: The Next Generation of Prevention, edited by Maurice J. Elias, PhD, and Joseph E. Zins, EdD (Vol. 19, No. 2, 2003). *"Current. . . . Provides a new perspective on this issue. . . . Of particular interest to those who work with middle school students." (Nancy Mullin-Rindler, MEd, Director, Project on Teasing and Bullying, Wellesley College Centers for Women)*

Computers in the Delivery of Special Education and Related Services: Developing Collaborative and Individualized Learning Environments, edited by Louis J. Kruger, PsyD (Vol. 17, No. 1/2, 2002). *"An excellent compendium. . . . The topics selected cover a broad conceptual spectrum, yet provide specific and useful information for the practitioner. A valuable resource for professionals at all levels. I highly recommend it." (David G. Gotthelf, PhD, Director of Student Services, Lincoln-Sudbury Regional School District, Massachusetts)*

Inclusion Practices with Special Needs Students: Theory, Research, and Application, edited by Steven I. Pfeiffer, PhD, ABPP, and Linda A. Reddy, PhD (Vol. 15, No. 1/2, 1999). *Provides a much needed and balanced perspective of the issues faced by educators committed to understanding how to best serve children with disabilities in schools.*

Emerging School-Based Approaches for Children with Emotional and Behavioral Problems: Research and Practice in Service Integration, edited by Robert J. Illback, PsyD, and C. Michael Nelson, EdD (Vol. 10, No. 2, and Vol. 11, No. 1/2, 1996). *"A stimulating and valuable contribution to the topic." (Donald K. Routh, PhD, Professor of Psychology, University of Miami)*

Educational Outcomes for Students with Disabilities, edited by James E. Ysseldyke, PhD, and Martha L. Thurlow (Vol. 9, No. 2, 1995). *"Clearly directed at teaching staff, psychologists, and other educationists but has relevance to all who work with children and young people with disabilities in schools of further education. . . . A useful book." (Physiotherapy)*

Promoting Student Success Through Group Interventions, edited by Joseph E. Zins, EdD, and Maurice J. Elias, PhD (Vol. 8, No. 1, 1994). *"Contains clear, concise, and practical descriptions of a variety of group interventions designed to promote students' success in school and life." (Social Work with Groups Newsletter)*

Promoting Success with At-Risk Students: Emerging Perspectives and Practical Approaches, edited by Louis J. Kruger, PsyD (Vol. 5, No. 3/4, 1990). *"Essential to professionals interested in new developments in the education of at-risk students, guidelines for implementation of approaches, and the prevention of student crises and discipline problems." (Virginia Child Protection Newsletter)*

Leadership and Supervision in Special Services: Promising Ideas and Practices, edited by Leonard C. Burrello, EdD, and David E. Greenburg, EdD (Vol. 4, No. 1/2, 1988). *A rich source of ideas for administrative personnel involved in the delivery of special educational programs and services to children with handicapping conditions.*

School-Based Affective and Social Interventions, edited by Susan G. Forman, PhD (Vol. 3, No. 3/4, 1988). *"Provides a valuable starting point for the psychologist, counselor, or other special service provider, special educator, regular classroom teacher, nurse, vice-principal, or other administrator who is willing to get involved in the struggle to help children and adolescents feel good about themselves and get along better in this world." (Journal of Pediatric Nursing)*

Facilitating Cognitive Development: International Perspectives, Programs, and Practices, edited by Milton S. Schwebel and Charles A. Maher, PsyD (Vol. 3, No. 1/2, 1986). *Experts discuss the vital aspects of programs and services that will facilitate cognitive development in children and adolescents.*

Emerging Perspectives on Assessment of Exceptional Children, edited by Randy Elliot Bennett, EdD, and Charles A. Maher, PsyD (Vol. 2, No. 2/3, 1986). *"Contains a number of innovative and promising approaches to the topic of assessment. It is an important addition to the rapidly changing field of special education and should be read by any individual who is interested in the assessment of exceptional children." (Journal of Psychological Assessment)*

Health Promotion in the Schools: Innovative Approaches to Facilitating Physical and Emotional Well-Being, edited by Joseph E. Zins, Donald I. Wagner, and Charles A. Maher, PsyD (Vol. 1, No. 3, 1985). *"Examines new approaches to promoting physical and emotional well-being in the schools. . . . A good introduction to new-style health education." (Curriculum Review)*

Microcomputers and Exceptional Children, edited by Randy Elliot Bennett, EdD, and Charles A. Maher, PsyD (Vol. 1, No. 1, 1984). *"This volume provides both the experienced and novice micro buff with a solid overview of the potential and real uses of the technology with exceptional students." (Alex Thomas, PhD, Port Clinton, Ohio)*

Bullying, Peer Harassment, and Victimization in the Schools: The Next Generation of Prevention has been co-published simultaneously as *Journal of Applied School Psychology*™, Volume 19, Number 2 2003.

Cover design by Jennifer M. Gaska

Library of Congress Cataloging-in-Publication Data

Elias, Maurice J. Bullying, peer harassment, and victimization in the schools / Maurice J. Elias, Joseph E. Zins.
    p. cm.
    Includes bibliographical references and index.
    ISBN 0-7890-2228-1 (alk. paper) – ISBN 0-7890-2229-X (pbk. : alk. paper)
    1. Bullying. 2. Aggressiveness in children. 3. Aggressiveness in adolescence. 4. School psychology. I. Zins, Joseph E. II. Title.
BF637.B85E45 2003
373.15′8–dc22
                                                                    2003015572

Bullying, Peer Harassment, and Victimization in the Schools: The Next Generation of Prevention

Maurice J. Elias, PhD
Joseph E. Zins, EdD
Editors

Bullying, Peer Harassment, and Victimization in the Schools: The Next Generation of Prevention has been co-published simultaneously as *Journal of Applied School Psychology*, Volume 19, Number 2 2003.

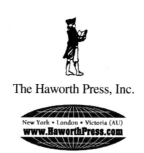

The Haworth Press, Inc.

New York • London • Victoria (AU)
www.HaworthPress.com

Indexing, Abstracting & Website/Internet Coverage

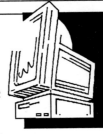

This section provides you with a list of major indexing & abstracting services. That is to say, each service began covering this periodical during the year noted in the right column. Most Websites which are listed below have indicated that they will either post, disseminate, compile, archive, cite or alert their own Website users with research-based content from this work. (This list is as current as the copyright date of this publication.)

Abstracting, Website/Indexing Coverage......... Year When Coverage Began

- *Australian Education Index <http://www.acer.edu.au>* 2000

- *Child Development Abstracts & Bibliography (in print & online)* ... 1985

- *CNPIEC Reference Guide: Chinese National Directory of Foreign Periodicals* 1995

- *Content Pages in Education* 1992

- *Education Digest* 1992

- *Educational Administration Abstracts (EAA)* 1991

- *e-psyche, LLC <http://www.e-psyche.net>* 2000

- *ERIC Clearinghouse on Counseling and Student Services (ERIC/CASS)* 1994

- *ERIC Clearinghouse on Rural Education & Small Schools* 1991

- *Exceptional Child Education Resources (ECER), (CD/ROM from SilverPlatter and hard copy)* 1985

(continued)

Special Bibliographic Notes related to special journal issues (separates) and indexing/abstracting:

- indexing/abstracting services in this list will also cover material in any "separate" that is co-published simultaneously with Haworth's special thematic journal issue or DocuSerial. Indexing/abstracting usually covers material at the article/chapter level.

- monographic co-editions are intended for either non-subscribers or libraries which intend to purchase a second copy for their circulating collections.

- monographic co-editions are reported to all jobbers/wholesalers/approval plans. The source journal is listed as the "series" to assist the prevention of duplicate purchasing in the same manner utilized for books-in-series.

- to facilitate user/access services all indexing/abstracting services are encouraged to utilize the co-indexing entry note indicated at the bottom of the first page of each article/chapter/contribution.

- this is intended to assist a library user of any reference tool (whether print, electronic, online, or CD-ROM) to locate the monographic version if the library has purchased this version but not a subscription to the source journal.

- individual articles/chapters in any Haworth publication are also available through the Haworth Document Delivery Service (HDDS).

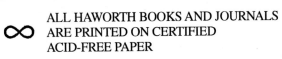

Bullying, Peer Harassment, and Victimization in the Schools: The Next Generation of Prevention

CONTENTS

ABOUT THE EDITORS

Maurice J. Elias, PhD, is Professor, Psychology Department, Rutgers University, and Co-Developer of the Social Decision Making/Social Problem Solving Project, named as a Model Program by the National Educational Goals Panel, and as a Promising Program by the U.S. Dept. of Education Expert Panel on Safe, Disciplined, and Drug-Free Schools. He is Leadership Team Vice Chair for the Collaborative for Academic, Social, and Emotional Learning (*www.CASEL.org*) and co-author of *Promoting Social and Emotional Learning: Guidelines for Educators* (ASCD, 1997). He is a member of the expert panel that advised the development of the *Early Warning Signs, Timely Response* book on violence prevention and subsequent materials, and he is the author of numerous books and articles on prevention. He is a past winner of the Lela Rowland Prevention Award and the Society for Community Research and Action's Distinguished Contribution to Practice award. Dr. Elias devotes his research and writing to the area of emotional intelligence in children, schools, and families. Recent books are *Emotionally Intelligent Parenting, Raising Emotionally Intelligent Teenagers: Guiding the Way for Compassionate, Committed, Courageous Adults* (Three Rivers Press/Random House, 2002) and *Engaging the Resistant Child Through Computers: A Manual for Social and Emotional Learning* (National Professional Resources, www.nprinc.com, 2001). New professional books include *Building Learning Communities with Character: How to Integrate Academic, Social, and Emotional Learning* (ASCD, 2002) and *EQ + IQ = Best Leadership Practices for Caring and Successful Schools* (Corwin Press, 2003).

Joseph E. Zins, EdD, is Professor in the College of Education at the University of Cincinnati and has nearly 30 years of applied experience. He is recognized nationally and internationally as an expert on individual and organizational consultation, social competence promotion, prevention, and psychological service delivery systems. Professor Zins has over 150 scientific publications and is past Editor of the multidisciplinary *Journal of Educational and Psychological Consultation.* Dr. Zins is a Fellow of the American Psychological Association, a member of the Leadership Team of the Collaborative for Academic, Social, and Emotional Learning (CASEL), and a former Secretary of the National Association of School Psychologists (NASP).

Bullying, Other Forms of Peer Harassment, and Victimization in the Schools: Issues for School Psychology Research and Practice

Maurice J. Elias

Rutgers University

Joseph E. Zins

University of Cincinnati

SUMMARY. Bullying and harassment are pervasive problems in our schools, affecting at least 70% of the student body. For years these behaviors have been overlooked, ignored, or viewed as part of "normal" development. However, we now know that these actions can have significant adverse effects on both perpetrators and victims. The research contained in this volume focuses primarily on the assessment and understanding of the most salient aspects of the problem, and the discussion thereby has substantial implications for intervention. Based on the contents, important directions for research and practice are identified. The article concludes with suggestions regarding the need to make changes in the culture and

Address correspondence to: Maurice J. Elias, Department of Psychology, Rutgers University, 53 Avenue E., Livingston Campus, Piscataway, NJ 08854-8040.

[Haworth co-indexing entry note]: "Bullying, Other Forms of Peer Harassment, and Victimization in the Schools: Issues for School Psychology Research and Practice." Elias, Maurice J., and Joseph E. Zins. Co-published simultaneously in *Journal of Applied School Psychology* (The Haworth Press, Inc.) Vol. 19, No. 2, 2003, pp. 1-5; and: *Bullying, Peer Harassment, and Victimization in the Schools: The Next Generation of Prevention* (ed: Maurice J. Elias, and Joseph E. Zins) The Haworth Press, Inc., 2003, pp. 1-5. Single or multiple copies of this article are available for a fee from The Haworth Document Delivery Service [1-800-HAWORTH, 9:00 a.m. - 5:00 p.m. (EST). E-mail address: docdelivery@haworthpress.com].

climate of our schools, using an expanded, ecological, and developmental perspective so these organizations are safe, caring, supportive places of academic, social, and emotional learning. *[Article copies available for a fee from The Haworth Document Delivery Service: 1-800-HAWORTH. E-mail address: <docdelivery@haworthpress.com> Website: <http://www.HaworthPress.com> © 2003 by The Haworth Press, Inc. All rights reserved.]*

KEYWORDS. Bullying, peer aggression, victimization, prevalence and normalization, social and emotional learning

Emerging research into the areas of bullying, peer sexual harassment, and other forms of student intimidation and threat in schools yields some remarkable and deeply disturbing convergences. The articles in this volume represent the early stages of a wave of ground-breaking work that will influence the direction of both researchers and practitioners for at least the next decade. From our perspective as psychologists involved in the school, clinical, and community psychology fields, as well as in our roles as members of the Leadership Team of the Collaborative for Academic, Social, and Emotional Learning (*www.CASEL.org*), the focus of this volume is long overdue.

A PERVASIVE AND SERIOUS ISSUE FOR SCHOOL MENTAL HEALTH AND ACADEMIC ACHIEVEMENT

Bullying and harassment are pervasive problems in our schools (Swearer & Cary, Nansel et al., and Holt & Espelage found 70% of the student body affected), and surprisingly large numbers of children are affected by sexual harassment (Young & Raffaele Mendez). As several of the articles indicate, bullying traditionally has been and continues to be overlooked, ignored, or viewed as a "normal" developmental behavior. Statements such as, "Boys will be boys," "She shouldn't dress like that if she doesn't want the attention," and "She shouldn't take that stuff, but give it right back," were and are made openly by supervising adults. Victims frequently are blamed, almost as if they were the perpetrators. However, we now know that even actions as common as teasing, "dissing," and shunning can have significant effects on perpetrators and victims and can result in missed school, poor grades, depression, low self-esteem, aggression, and suicide. And, as Holt and Espelage reported, those who experience multiple forms of victimization are impacted especially strongly.

The research presented in this volume significantly contributes to the literature. It focuses primarily on assessment and understanding of the nuances of the problem, and thereby has substantial implications for intervention. A number of the studies address middle school issues and involve multiethnic populations, including those from Canada and Europe, as well as within the United States, and they also cross socioeconomic lines and take a longitudinal perspective. In addition, other articles clearly integrate peer sexual harassment and dating-related aggression into discussions that previously have been predominantly oriented to traditional views of bullying and peer intimidation, and accordingly serve to expand our knowledge of the issues.

Developmental studies are especially important because they begin to allow some inferences about directionality of effects. A persistent question, for example, is the extent to which pre-existing psychological difficulties lead to victimization, which in turn leads to poor school outcomes, versus victimization leading to psychological destabilization, which then results in deteriorating academic functioning. Data from Paul and Cillessen, as well as Goldbaum et al. and Nansel et al., suggest that the latter is a more prevalent model than the former. That is, victimization, as well as being a bully-victim, seems highly deleterious to children. Indeed, those who cease being victimized have outcomes more similar to those who were never victims than to those who remain in that status. Future research needs to understand much more about the conditions under which victim status is changed.

DIRECTIONS FOR RESEARCH AND PRACTICE

Among the important directions for research and practice that this collection of articles suggests are the following:

- We must continue to take a more differentiated and developmental perspective on bullies, victims, and bully-victims. The continuity of bullying and victimization over time and across different school settings, as well as changes in status on the part of a given student, are salient factors in understanding risk.
- Victims are truly victimized by what happens to them. Their outcomes are worse than those of the bullies. Further, there is no doubt that some bullies, perhaps as many as half, enjoy positive status, not only from peers but from teachers. Those victims who then become bullies are a group at the early stages of being understood by researchers; their situation may well be the most problematic of all the subgroups, although some data suggest that continued victimization produces the worst outcomes.

- Methodologically, it is important to recognize that different data sources may yield different conclusions about who is perpetrating and receiving harassment. Teachers, other students, and the self-report of the child reflect distinctive perspectives which may or may not converge, for reasons that Graham et al. explore in detail.
- Research must continue to examine differential effects as a function of gender, ethnic and cultural group, SES, and type of school. Information about the latter is relatively lacking in the research base thus far, other than confirming the prevalence of significant peer harassment across a wide range of school contexts. Findings by both Strohmeier and Spiel and by Graham et al. indicate that subgroups can be selected out for greater victimization, or at least a lower degree of social integration.

LORD OF THE FLIES *REVISITED IN OUR SCHOOLS?*

Disquieting, however, is what the data suggest about life in schools. It would appear as if there is a culture (indeed, it is too prevalent to call a subculture but might even approach a "norm") of intimidation in schools that does not emerge in discussions of school reform and school change, and also does not surface as a primary organizational concern of school psychologists. The accumulated research, in this volume and elsewhere, suggests a very serious and pressing need to examine peer culture in schools and the roles of adults in inadvertently and often unknowingly creating and enabling its negative elements.

Consider this quote: "Girls who physically fight back may not only be punished by the boys who attack them, but unfairly and unevenly by school authorities. The narrative of girls who are harassed and who respond actively to that harassment are filled with stories of unjust punishment" (Rodkin & Fischer, p. 190). This report represents a highly complex situation, since other data suggest that those who fight back are headed for especially poor outcomes, and many bullies are seen as popular and admirable by both peers and teachers. Also think about Swearer and Cary's data on where most bullying takes place: classrooms, hallways, after school, gym, and recess. In four of these five contexts, adults should be providing supervision and *de facto* protection.

Is this *The Lord of the Flies* revisited? In the absence of adult structure, are children creating a society based on social power? Is the prevalence of bullying and harassment a sign of how many students feel disconnected from the subculture of academic, athletic, and artistic performance successes in schools and the star culture that fuels each? Debates about school safety and legislative and programmatic anti-bullying interventions would do well to be informed by the findings of the research presented in this volume. This research speaks to the role of adults in schools, the interpersonal structure of school safety, and the pervasive and harmful nature of the trends observed. All this has happened on the watch of school psychologists; so what shall the response be? Perhaps a warning from Seymour Sarason in *The Culture of the Schools and the Problem of Change* (1982) is in order. Focusing on individuals and programs rather than the culture and climate of schools is the road too often traveled. Only by taking an expanded, ecological, and developmental perspective is the field likely to make major and lasting contributions to research and practice around how our schools can become more caring, supportive, safe, and effective places of academic, social, and emotional learning.

REFERENCE

Sarason, S. B. (1982). *The culture of the schools and the problem of change* (2nd ed.). Boston: Allyn & Bacon.

The Mental Health Professional's Role in Understanding, Preventing, and Responding to Student Sexual Harassment

Ellie L. Young

Brigham Young University

Linda M. Raffaele Mendez

University of South Florida

SUMMARY. Sexual harassment is a common experience in today's schools. A majority of secondary students report experiencing sexual harassment at school, with many reporting that they experienced it in elementary school as well. This article provides mental health professionals working in schools with an understanding of sexual harassment so that they can be proactive in responding to harassment and developing effective interventions. The first section of the article provides a working definition, including examples of various situations that may be encountered, and distinctions between sexual and gender harassment. Subsequent sections address gender and ethnicity issues, developmental

---

Address correspondence to: Ellie L. Young, Department of Counseling Psychology and Special Education, 340-N MCKB, Brigham Young University, Provo, UT 84602 (E-mail: ellie_young@byu.edu).

[Haworth co-indexing entry note]: "The Mental Health Professional's Role in Understanding, Preventing, and Responding to Student Sexual Harassment." Young, Ellie L., and Linda M. Raffaele Mendez. Co-published simultaneously in *Journal of Applied School Psychology* (The Haworth Press, Inc.) Vol. 19, No. 2, 2003, pp. 7-23; and: *Bullying, Peer Harassment, and Victimization in the Schools: The Next Generation of Prevention* (ed: Maurice J. Elias, and Joseph E. Zins) The Haworth Press, Inc., 2003, pp. 7-23. Single or multiple copies of this article are available for a fee from The Haworth Document Delivery Service [1-800-HAWORTH, 9:00 a.m. - 5:00 p.m. (EST). E-mail address: docdelivery@haworthpress.com].

factors, special concerns related to gay and lesbian students, and pertinent legal issues (including a brief review of recent court cases). The article concludes with specific primary, secondary, and tertiary prevention strategies that can be used to address sexual harassment in schools. *[Article copies available for a fee from The Haworth Document Delivery Service: 1-800-HAWORTH. E-mail address: <docdelivery@haworthpress.com> Website: <http://www.HaworthPress.com> © 2003 by The Haworth Press, Inc. All rights reserved.]*

KEYWORDS. Sexual harassment, mental health professional, intervention strategies, legal issues in sexual harassment, school climate

Sexual harassment is unwanted and unwelcome behavior that interferes with a student's participation in an educational program. Sexual harassment can include verbal comments, nonverbal communication, or physical contact. Unwanted sexual advances or requests for sexual favors are considered sexual harassment. To be identified as sexual harassment, the behavior must be either implicitly or explicitly sexual and be perceived by the recipient as undesirable (Paludi, 1997; Stein, 1999).

Sexual harassment is a common experience for the majority of today's secondary school students in the United States. Recently, 81% of secondary students reported experiencing sexual harassment during their educational careers (American Association of University Women [AAUW], 2001). Approximately one-third of students reported first experiencing sexual harassment before sixth grade. Sexual harassment is not something that happens just to girls: 79% of boys and 83% of girls reported being sexually harassed at school, although boys and girls experience sexual harassment quite differently. Most incidents of sexual harassment occur in public places in schools, such as classrooms, hallways, and cafeterias (AAUW, 2001). Sexual harassment has become pervasive to the extent that it is considered part of adolescent culture (Lee, Croninger, Linn, & Chen, 1996).

Mental health professionals' understanding of human development and behavior, emotional health, and school organization provides a foundation to become effectively proactive and responsive in addressing sexual harassment issues. Their training and work assignments facilitate their role as an advocate and leader for anti-harassment efforts. They easily can become the point person for anti-harassment efforts. This article first presents a working definition, including specific examples of sexual harassment. A brief section clarifies the distinctions between sexual and gender harassment. Next, current research about prevalence, gender, and ethnicity issues is reviewed. In addition, a brief integration of developmental and sexual harassment is discussed. A legal history is included to assist mental health professionals when they are asked to consult with school administrators on these issues. Finally, several levels of effective prevention and intervention strategies are presented. With this foundational knowledge, psychologists, counselors, and social workers will be better equipped to be advocates for and participants in successful intervention and prevention of sexual harassment.

DEFINING SEXUAL HARASSMENT

The legal definition of sexual harassment is "unwelcome sexual advances, requests for sexual favors, sexually motivated physical conduct or other verbal or physical conduct" that limits a student's participation in an educational program (U.S. Department of Education, Office for Civil Rights and National Association of Attorneys General, 1999, p. 17). The context of the behavior, the difference in status and power of the victim and perpetrator, as well as the impact of the behavior must be considered. Although this definition of sexual harassment is quite succinct, in practice, defining and identifying sexual harassment can be quite challenging, especially for students.

In contrast to sexual harassment, good-natured teasing and flirting tend to be mutually acceptable, enjoyable, and pleasant, and both parties participate willingly. When sexual harassment occurs the targets may feel threatened, embarrassed, fearful, or self-conscious. Power and intimidation are inherent in sexual harassment. Victims of sexual harassment experience an absence of choice and control, and perpetrators communicate a sense of hostility (AAUW, 2001, Levy & Paludi, 2002; Stein & Sjostrom, 1994). Distinguishing between normal teasing and unwanted harassment is a social skill that requires accurately perceiving others' feelings and intentions (Goldstein, 1999; Elias et al., 1997).

At the other end of the continuum, sexual assault and rape would be extreme forms of sexual harassment, if the context is in the workplace or an educational setting. Legally, sexual harassment does not occur in personal or private relationships, the context is an employment or school environment where a person with power abuses that power to coerce some one because of his or her sex. The most common forms of sexual harassment, such as sexist comments or gestures, do not have legal consequences when they are experienced to lesser extents. However, rape is a criminal offense, which has distinctly different legal implications (Levi & Paludi, 2002; Paludi & Barickman, 1998).

Quid pro quo and hostile environment have been the most commonly discussed forms of sexual harassment (Shoop & Edwards, 1994). Quid pro quo literally means "you do something for me and I'll do something for you." It also can include threats to avoid harm rather than achieving any gain. This type of harassment happens when a person with authority, such as a teacher or a coach, demands a sexual favor in return for some educational benefit or avoidance of harm. He or she may request a sexual favor in return for a higher grade or a position on the varsity soccer team (Paludi, 1997). Quid pro quo harassment also can occur among students. A student editor might threaten a student reporter to perform sexual acts in order to keep her or his coveted assignments (see Stein, 1999).

A hostile environment exists when sexual teasing, insulting, touching, or other unwanted sexual behavior is pervasive, persistent, and severe to the extent that students' ability to participate in or benefit from an educational program is denied (U.S. Department of Education, 2001). One incidence of teasing or similar behavior generally will not constitute legally significant sexual harassment. The behavior may violate the school's policy, be offensive and insulting, and require school discipline, but not have legal consequences. Legal action is a result of significant and severe harassment that impedes a student's participation in an educational program (Paludi, 1997).

Sexual harassment can take many forms. The most common types reported by secondary school students include both sexual comments and jokes and physical actions, such as being touched, grabbed, pinched, or brushed against in a sexual way (AAUW, 2001). Sexually harassing comments can include being persistently called "babe" or "sweetheart," sexual or gender insults, or remarks about specific body parts. Leering, displaying pornography, writing sexual graffiti, and rumor mongering have been legally identified as sexual harassment (Shoop & Hayhow, 1994; U.S. Department of Education, 2002).

The impact of the behavior rather than the intent of the behavior determines if sexual harassment has occurred (Paludi, 1997). For example, if a girl repeatedly blows kisses at a boy or pinches his buttocks several times to the extent that the young man is uncomfortable or irritated, her behavior has created a hostile environment, even though her intention was to develop a dating relationship. Perpetrators and their targets often have different perspectives about the intent of the harassing behavior. Those who harass may perceive their behavior as flattering, inoffensive teasing, or harmless touching, while the target finds it unpleasant, awkward, or humiliating (Layman, 1994). Using the impact rather than the intent standard of determining if sexual harassment has occurred can be problematic because the rights of the accused may not be considered. To address this issue, those investigating the claim determine if a "reasonable woman" or "reasonable man" experiencing the alleged harassment would find the behavior offensive. Using the same gender perspective as the victim is imperative because males and females tend to have different perceptions of harassing behavior (Levy & Paludi, 2002).

Some have expressed concern that the well-intentioned hug from a teacher to a student will be construed as sexual harassment. The U.S. Department of Education's Office for Civil Rights (OCR) guidelines clearly indicate that not all physical contact between teachers and students or between students is sexual harassment. For example, comforting a child with a skinned knee is not sexual harassment, and neither is a coach hugging a player after the player has made a goal. Physical contact between students that is nonsexual, such as practicing a sports maneuver, also does not constitute sexual harassment. However, nonsexual contact may be interpreted as sexual harassment if it occurs repeatedly and under inappropriate circumstances (U.S. Department of Education, 2001).

GAY AND LESBIAN ISSUES

The harsh and cruel incidents of harassment and bullying reported by gay, lesbian, bisexual, transgender, or questioning students are more likely to be gender harassment rather than sexual harassment (Human Rights Watch, 2001). Gender harassment includes behaviors that are verbally or physically aggressive, intimidating, or hostile but are not sexual or a sexual proposition (Stein, 1999). In contrast to sexual harassment, gender harassment focuses on behaviors that target a person because of his or her sexual orientation or behaviors that do not fit socio-cultural norms for the victim's gender (U.S. Department of Education, 2001). The OCR has provided two examples to clarify sexual and gender harassment. If a female student who is a lesbian sexually propositions another female student to the extent that a hostile environment is created, a legally significant occurrence of sexual harassment has occurred. If a female student harasses another female student about her sexual orientation, gender harassment has occurred.

When students are harassed or bullied because of their sexual orientation, the Equal Protection Clause of the Fourteenth Amendment of the U.S. Constitution provides a safeguard. Generally, legal issues arise when harassment of sexual minority students has been ignored by school authority figures. In 1996, a federal court awarded a Wisconsin student, Jamie Nabozny, over $900,000 for the harassment he endured when school administrators repeatedly ignored his complaints of severe harassment based on his sexual identity. One administrator allegedly told Jamie that he should get used to the torment because he was so openly gay. In this case, cause is not the issue; harassment in any form, for any reason is unacceptable (Henning-Stout, James, & Macintosh, 2000;

Stein, 1999; U.S. Department of Education, Office for Civil Rights and National Association of Attorneys General, 1999).

PREVALENCE OF SEXUAL HARASSMENT

One of the most comprehensive investigations of the prevalence of sexual harassment in schools was commissioned by the American Association of University Women in 1993 (AAUW, 1993) and then repeated in 2001. The questions on the survey related only to sexual harassment at school or school-related activities, and sexual harassment was defined as "unwanted and unwelcome sexual behavior that interferes with your life. Sexual harassment is not behaviors that you like or want" (AAUW, 2001, p. 2). The percentage of students reporting sexual harassment at school did not change from 1993 to 2001. The most dramatic change occurred in the students' awareness of their schools' sexual harassment policy: there was a 40% increase in students reporting their awareness of a school sexual harassment policy. Although it appears that students are more aware of school policies against sexual harassment, this alone does not seem to be decreasing the prevalence of sexual harassment. In fact, educating students about policy may actually increase the reports of harassment because it normalizes reporting offensive behavior (Brooks & Perot, 1991). Increasing awareness of sexual harassment policies may be a necessary but insufficient condition for decreasing sexual harassment.

Although boys (79%) and girls (83%) reported experiencing comparable frequencies of sexual harassment, these data can be misleading. Girls reported experiencing harassment somewhat more frequently, experiencing more severe types of harassment, and having more negative emotional reactions to harassment than boys. When girls experienced harassment, they were more likely than boys to report being upset by it and feeling self-conscious, embarrassed, afraid, and less self-assured. Girls indicated that sexual harassment contributes to feelings of shame: "dirty–like a piece of trash," "like a second-class citizen," and "sick to my stomach" (AAUW, 2001, p. 36). Girls also were more likely than boys to be harassed by a school-related adult, which tends to be more severe than student-to-student harassment. Girls were more likely to report sexual harassment to authority figures (Stein, 1999: AAUW, 2001). In contrast, when boys report sexual harassment, Stein (1999) suggested that boys may experience a second victimization because attention from girls generally is viewed as an honor or rite of passage. Boys who complain about inappropriate sexual attention from girls go against cultural norms.

Ethnicity also plays a role in what types of harassment students experience and how students report feeling about it. White males are more likely to be called gay or to have their clothes pulled at or down in a sexual way. Hispanic males are more likely to be the brunt of sexual jokes, comments, gestures, or looks. When young Black females and males experience harassment, they report being less affected than either White or Hispanic students. White females are more likely to be the targets of rumors and are more likely to be called a lesbian. Black females are more likely to report being touched, grabbed, or pinched in a sexual way or to have their clothing pulled at in a sexual manner (AAUW, 2001). Although these statements are quite general, they illustrate how ethnicity may play a role in how an individual experiences and responds to sexual harassment. In addition, it encourages the use of a multicultural perspective in understanding sexual harassment or developing interventions.

Further analysis of the data from the AAUW (1993) survey on sexual harassment revealed that almost 75% of students who indicated that they were victims of sexual harassment also claimed that they had been a perpetrator of sexual harassment at least once, which is comparable to the 53% of students reporting being both a victim and a bully in the bullying literature (Haynie et al., 2001). However, because the sexual harassment data are not longitudinal, determining whether victimization or perpetration came first is not possible. These findings have important implications for preventing and responding to sexual harassment. When schools adopt only a punish-the-perpetrator model of responding to sexual harassment, the cultural context of sexual harassment is not integrated into the conceptualization of the problem. Effective interventions will be aimed at creating an inclusive and respectful school climate (Lee et al., 1996).

DEVELOPMENTAL ISSUES

When sexual harassment policies are applied rigidly and student developmental issues are disregarded, the children involved are not well-served. For example, in 1996, a six-year-old boy kissed a girl in his class and was accused of sexual harassment. Common sense and understanding of human development would lead most educators to the conclusion that young students or students with developmental delays may not understand the complexities and sexual content of adolescent and adult sexual harassment. However, caution is warranted in interpreting not only the teasing or harassing behaviors but the impact of these behaviors among young children. Sexual harassment in early elementary school frequently is viewed as just teasing, bullying, or normal childhood play. However, this perception can be at odds with federal mandates. Sexual harassment can occur among elementary students, but the victim's perceptions about the interaction and the context of the behavior need to be considered (Stein, 1999).

As students move from elementary school to junior high or middle school, several factors contribute to increased incidence of sexual harassment. As early adolescents experience the physical changes of puberty, move from same-sex to mixed-sex peer groups, and begin to experience sexual feelings, sexually harassing behavior may be an attempt to explore their sexuality and to realize new ways of interacting with their peers. Within this age group, the distinction between flirting and sexual harassment may not be evident to many students (Craig, Pepler, Connolly, & Henderson, 2001). Other developmental issues associated with sexual harassment include the increased likelihood that either males or females who experience puberty earlier than their peers may be more likely to be targets of sexual harassment because early maturation is a highly salient characteristic during early adolescence and is typically an effective means of creating distress for students in this age group. Early developers and their peers may not have attained the cognitive and emotional resources to deal with these complicated issues. Their still-developing social skills may not correspond to their physical development (Craig et al., 2001).

Mental health professionals' understanding of child and adolescent development can help administrators develop reasonable responses to sexual harassment claims. Through assessment, observations, and interviews, psychologists, counselors, and social workers can assist in determining developmentally appropriate interventions and disciplinary actions. Professionals need to attend not only to developmental issues but also to a child's disability, especially if that child has been identified with an emotional or behavioral disability.

PROCEDURAL AND LEGAL ISSUES

The legal mandate that addresses sexual harassment of students is Title IX of the Educational Amendments of 1972, which applies to all educational institutions receiving federal funding. Title IX prohibits discrimination in educational programs based on sex; and sexual harassment has been determined by courts to be a form of sex discrimination (Stein, 1999). Under Title IX, lawsuits are brought against educational institutions rather than individuals. However, a student may have recourse against the individual perpetrator on the basis of other federal or state law (Layman, 1994). Both females and males are protected by Title IX (U.S. Department of Education, 2002).

Title IX mandates that schools take three actions to address sexual discrimination and therefore sexual harassment. First, school districts must have a policy stating that they do not discriminate on the basis of sex in determining participation in any of their educational programs (Stone, 2000). Schools are not required to have a sexual harassment policy that is separate from their sexual discrimination policy, but this is recommended (Webb, Hunnicutt, & Metha, 1997). Second, school districts must have published guidelines on sex discrimination and inform employees and students of this policy. Third, this policy must include a grievance procedure to address complaints. If a school district fails to meet these three stipulations, the district may be found in violation of Title IX, and its federal funding could be threatened (Layman, 1994).

While there are approximately two dozen court cases that have influenced sexual harassment policy, there are several that merit the attention of school-based professionals. The first case that held a school monetarily liable for sexual harassment was *Franklin v. Gwinnett County (GA) Public Schools.* In the 20-year existence of Title IX, this was the first time that a school district was held liable for compensatory damages because of failure to provide an educational setting free from sexual discrimination. In this case, a male teacher had sexual intercourse with a female student three times on campus. The administration arranged the resignation of the teacher, and no further action against the teacher was taken. The courts decided that the young woman had experienced sexual discrimination, and she was granted compensatory damages (Stein, 1999; Layman, 1994).

Some school districts have questioned their liability to protect students from other sexually harassing students. In May 1999, the Supreme Court clarified that school districts can be held liable for student-to-student harassment if the school knew about it but did not take reasonable steps to stop it. In the case of *Davis v. Monroe County Board of Education*, a male classmate seated next to a fifth-grade girl harassed her over a period of five months by grabbing her breasts and crotch, using sexual and crude language, and rubbing his body against hers (Stein, 1999). Incidents were reported by the child to her mother, who in turn reported the incidents to her daughter's teacher and the building principal. Only after three months were the children's desks moved. The young woman's grades dropped significantly, and a suicide note was discovered by her father. The sexual harassment did not stop until the parents filed a complaint with the sheriff's office and charged the young man with sexual battery, to which he plead guilty. Mrs. Davis then filed a sexual discrimination suit against the school under Title IX. The Supreme Court favored Mrs. Davis, explaining that its decision was influenced by the school's intentional lack of concern for the welfare of the young woman (Stein, 1999).

The Davis ruling clarified that liability for student-to-student harassment can be claimed only when the school has been "deliberately indifferent to sexual harassment, of which the recipient [of federal funding] has actual knowledge" (Biskupic, 1999, p. A.1). The guidance given by OCR (U.S. Department of Education, 2001) succinctly states, "If harassment has occurred, doing nothing is always the wrong response" (p. iii). OCR recognizes that schools cannot micro-manage students' behavior or propensity toward sexual harassment. However, OCR does expect school districts to respond to sexual harassment when they know about it or when they reasonably should have known about it. A response indicating that the student "asked for it" or that "it was just a joke" has been considered blatantly insufficient by OCR (Layman, 1994; U.S. Department of Education, 2001).

PRIMARY, SECONDARY, AND TERTIARY PREVENTION STRATEGIES

This section examines three levels of prevention aimed at decreasing sexual harassment: (a) primary prevention (e.g., initiatives targeted at all students and faculty to prevent or decrease occurrences of sexual harassment); (b) secondary prevention (e.g., initiatives targeted toward those who are at risk for engaging in sexual harassment of others or who are at risk of being the target of sexual harassment); and (c) tertiary prevention (e.g., initiatives and interventions that focus on perpetrators and their targets after repeated harassment already has occurred, and that aim to prevent its further recurrence and to minimize the negative impact).

Primary prevention. Educators are recognizing that primary prevention of sexual harassment in schools is rooted in a school's overall culture and climate (Stein, 1995; U.S. Department of Education, Office for Civil Rights and National Association of Attorneys General, 1999). A recent government publication focusing on protecting students from harassment and hate crimes noted "a growing consensus among educators that the best way to protect students from harassment is to establish a secure environment that expects appropriate behavior and promotes tolerance, sensitivity to others' views, and cooperative interactions among students" (U.S. Department of Education, Office for Civil Rights and National Association of Attorneys General, 1999, p. 8). Mental health professionals in the schools are key players in assisting administrators to understand the importance of school climate in sexual harassment prevention, to identify the most effective ways to measure school climate, and to develop interventions to improve school climate.

Some of the most important climate-related questions that school personnel can ask themselves are: Do staff, students, and parents perceive an atmosphere of mutual respect and understanding at their school? Does the school climate reflect an appreciation for differences and diversity? What is the level of support among administrators and staff in implementing the sexual harassment policy? A school climate survey can be an effective way to answer these and similar questions, and several are available for use in the schools (Lehr & Christenson, 2002). Overall school climate is key to sexual harassment prevention efforts because in schools where there is little caring, respect, or trust between teachers and students, it is doubtful that students will approach school adults for help in resolving problems. Excellent suggestions for improving overall school climate with regard to appreciation of racial, cultural, and other forms of diversity can be accessed at http://www.ed.gov/pubs/Harassment/climate1.html and http://www.CASEL.org.

In addition to considering overall school climate, mental health professionals can directly assess the perceptions of sexual harassment at their schools by using separate teacher, parent, and student surveys targeted at sexual harassment (see AAUW (2002) and United States Department of Education, Office for Civil Rights and National Association of Attorneys General (1999), Appendix B, p. 111). Publicly observed or survey reported sexual harassment is likely to be just the tip of the iceberg. In many schools, the majority of sexual harassment will go unreported and unidentified. These surveys can identify "hot spots" or create environmental maps to determine places in schools that are most troublesome.

Parents have many roles to play in addressing sexual harassment. They can and should be included in the school climate survey or other surveys about sexual harassment. Including parents in sexual harassment educational activities increases their awareness of the issues, which in turn helps them to be better advocates for their children and ensure that schools are safe places for children. Parents can help their children practice assertiveness skills and reporting harassing behaviors. Creating and maintaining effective communication between students and parents may be one of the most effective measures of dealing with sexual harassment (AAUW, 2002). Mental health professionals can refer parents to the materials from AAUW (2002) that identify specific activities to help parents to take the initiative in addressing these issues with their children and the schools.

As stated earlier, Title IX requires only that a school district have a published sex discrimination policy and a grievance procedure. However, best practices dictate that the policy contains a range of actions that could be taken when sexual harassment is substantiated. Mental health professionals should provide guidance to administrators in selecting targeted, age-appropriate responses for violating the policy. Depending on the severity, responses can range from providing education about sexual harassment and its effects on victims to more punitive responses, such as suspension or expulsion (Kopels & Dupper, 1999). Rather than touting a "zero tolerance" policy, the administrative response to sexual harassment should consider the age of the perpetrator and the target, as well as the nature and severity of the behavior. Using functional behavioral assessment strategies will ensure that positive behavioral interventions are designed to meet the student's specific needs.

Mental health professionals also can assist administrators to address the needs of the victim in the school's sexual harassment policy (Kopels & Dupper, 1999). A statement assuring the confidentiality of complaints should be included in the policy (Webb et al., 1997). The policy also should include pre-established guidelines for providing assistance to targets of sexual harassment, such as meeting with a peer support group or counselor at school. Finally, students should be assured that retaliation for making a complaint is not acceptable. If changes to a student's schedule are necessary, changes to the perpetrator's (rather than the victim's) schedule should be considered in addition to increased supervision where the harassment occurred (Shoop & Edwards, 1994). To help targets of sexual harassment feel more comfortable when making a complaint, the policy should stipulate that sexual harassment reports can be made to either a male or female official. Sexual harassment complaints should include written documentation of what happened, when, and who witnessed the events. Excellent examples of complaint forms are found in the new AAUW (2002) publication.

To ensure that the policy is effectively implemented, school personnel need training to identify sexual harassment and to intervene when they observe sexual harassment or when sexual harassment is reported to them. This training must be concrete and detailed; case studies may be useful. Role-plays may be especially effective in helping school adults become more comfortable in this role (Stein, 1993). This training also should include descriptions of the legal and emotional consequences of sexual harassment. All school adults (including paraprofessionals, bus drivers, cafeteria workers, and custodians) need to have the opportunity to clarify their own values, attitudes, and experiences about sexual harassment (Strauss, 1988). During the training school adults must be encouraged to model behavior at school that avoids sexual references, innuendoes, and jokes (AAUW, 2002). Notably, even with adequate training in how the policy is to be implemented, if there is insufficient staff buy-in or administrative support, it is unlikely the policy will be enforced and incorporated into the school culture.

When conducting training programs with students, their cognitive and emotional maturity must be carefully considered (e.g., elementary school students will need more concrete examples than high school students), and the trainer must be able to establish an atmosphere of trust among the students so that their feelings can be dealt with openly and honestly (Paludi & Barickman, 1998). Additionally, inviting others (e.g., parents, school board members) to participate in the training can help to ensure support outside of the classroom for students and teachers (Paludi & Barickman, 1998). Keeping males and females together ensures that all students receive consistent messages and communicates that both boys and girls can be targets of sexual harassment (Shoop & Edwards, 1994).

Notably, many professionals are already involved in building-level or district-wide primary prevention activities focused on increasing cultural sensitivity, tolerance of individual differences, and the development of pro-social behaviors. Consultants often train teachers, who then implement the curriculum in the classroom (e.g., Knoff & Batsche, 1995). In conjunction with these existing programs, folding in a sexual harassment curriculum may be a reasonable approach. Incorporating sexual harassment training into already existing social skills or character education initiatives may help to reduce the ecological intrusiveness of the training and increase teacher acceptance of the intervention (see Witt, 1986). Elias et al. (1997) offer specific guidelines for social and emotional learning programs that can be applied to sexual harassment prevention programs.

Because little empirical research exists on the efficacy of sexual-harassment education in the schools, school personnel are left to choose a curriculum that appears educationally sound and that meets the needs of their students and teachers. Those choosing or developing the curriculum should be aware that students' perceptions of using assemblies or classroom videos were not positive (AAUW, 2001). Students want adults to *talk* to them about these issues. A discussion-oriented curriculum entitled *Flirting or Hurting* was developed for grades 6-12 (Stein & Sjostrom, 1994). Additionally, fairly concrete curriculum, with different lesson plans for elementary and secondary students, can be found in the appendix of Paludi and Barickman (1998). A program developed by the Minnesota Department of Education (1993) for grades K-3 and 4-6 also provides an excellent approach to teaching respect and tolerance to younger age groups

Secondary prevention. Secondary prevention of sexual harassment targets those who are at-risk for experiencing sexual harassment as either a victim or a perpetrator. Although predicting with accuracy who is at-risk for engaging in sexual harassment is difficult, it is known that students who may be at greater risk include early maturing students and gay, lesbian, bisexual, or transgender students (Craig et al., 2001; Human Rights Watch, 2001). Other students targeted for intervention may be students who make inappropriate comments or gestures. For example, if a student makes offensive comments about girls' or boys' bodies during an in-class discussion (which often are humorous to other students but may be ignored by the teacher), the student is likely expressing an underlying attitude about others that also is reflected in other inappropriate behaviors outside the classroom. Teachers often know who these students are but are not aware of how to respond to them. Targeting these students for intervention and not just disciplinary action is key.

Teachers who notice students being teased, bullied, or harassed (even if the student does not report the behavior) should guide these students to school resources so that they can increase their skills in responding to harassment. Perpetrators also should be referred for intervention. Another important component includes training students who observe harassing behaviors not just to ignore what they see but to report the behavior to someone who can provide assistance. Shoop and Edwards (1994) offer a number of suggestions for teaching students how to be assertive and to document when they experience harassment. Readers are referred to Goldstein (1999) for ideas on intervening specifically with perpetrators of sexual harassment.

Tertiary prevention. The primary difference between tertiary prevention and secondary prevention entails initiatives that are focused on the most serious and chronic incidences of harassment. In this case, school personnel must know how to respond when a student engages in serious acts of sexual harassment or demonstrates a chronic pattern of such behavior. Additionally, they must know how to respond to and assist students with a pattern of victimization at school. Chronic perpetration of sexual harassment should be handled using a combination of disciplinary and educational interventions. Disciplinary actions may include exclusionary responses, such as suspension or expulsion in severe situations.

Exclusionary discipline techniques serve to protect other students from inappropriate behavior and send a message that such behaviors will not be tolerated, but they do not address the underlying issues that led to the behavior in the first place (Raffaele Mendez, Knoff, & Ferron, 2002). In the case of sexual harassment, students who show repeated disregard for the rights of others should have opportunities to learn skills for treating others with respect and for appreciating diversity. Mental health professionals can provide assistance to these students and their families by gathering additional information to determine which community and school resources may best meet their needs.

When sexual harassment is reported to a school adult, a critical first step is for the adult to listen and be responsive to the student's concerns and emotions. Title IX requires that school adults who have knowledge of sexual harassment report it to school officials who have the responsibility to investigate the claim and take corrective action. Additionally, Stone (2000) notes that OCR promotes protection of the confidentiality of the target of sexual harassment. The name of the victim need not be revealed if she or he would prefer to remain anonymous. This is true even if failure to identify the target would significantly impair the investigation of the alleged harassment. If the target does not wish to be identified, others who witnessed the harassment may be interviewed. It may, however, be necessary in cases where the victim's physical safety is threatened to reveal his or her identity so that the investigation can be pursued expediently. Additionally, staff should inform students that information about sexual harassment may need to be reported to the student's parents (Stone, 2000).

Finally, students who have experienced sexual harassment need to regain a sense of security and trust. This may be accomplished in a variety of ways, including peer support groups at school, individual counseling either at school or in the community, and opportunities for students who have experienced harassment to help other students understand its impact or assist with their recovery. Protection from retaliation is a part of regaining a sense of security. When working with groups of victims in a peer support group, group leaders should be aware of inadvertently reinforcing the victim role. Group leaders can help students who have experienced repeated victimization develop skills in assertion and personal power rather than focusing exclusively on the students' experiences as victims.

CONCLUSION

Mental health professionals working in the schools can do much to address sexual harassment. We have examined a working definition of sexual harassment, gender and ethnicity issues, developmental factors, and special concerns related to gay and lesbian students. We also have offered an overview of legislation and case law related to sexual harassment in schools. Additionally, we have discussed specific primary, secondary, and tertiary prevention strategies to be considered. We consider the area of primary prevention to be particularly important. Greater emphasis must be placed on developing respect and appreciation for diversity. Within this realm, school psychologists, counselors, and social workers can assist other educators in assessing school climate; developing comprehensive, developmentally sensitive sexual harassment policies; and designing effective training for students and staff in this area. Such efforts are likely to substantially reduce sexual harassment and lead to a safer, more comfortable, and more respectful learning environment for all students.

REFERENCES

American Association of University Women. (1993). *Hostile hallways: The AAUW survey on sexual harassment in America's schools.* Washington, DC: Author.
American Association of University Women. (2001). *Hostile hallways: Bullying, teasing, and sexual harassment in school.* Washington, DC: Author.

American Association of University Women. (2002). *Harassment-free hallways: How to stop sexual harassment in schools.* Washington, DC: Author.

Biskupic, K. (1999, May 25). *Davis v. Monroe County Board of Education et al. The Washington Post,* pp. A1:1.

Brooks, L. & Perot, A. R. (1991). Reporting sexual harassment: Exploring a predictive model. *Psychology of Women, 15,* 31-47.

Craig, W. M., Pepler, D., Connolly, J., & Henderson, K. (2001). Developmental context of peer harassment in early adolescence: The role of puberty and the peer group. In J. Juvonen & S. Graham (Eds.), *Peer harassment in school: The plight of the vulnerable and victimized* (pp. 242-261). New York: Guilford Press.

Elias, M. J., Zins, J. E., Weissberg, R. P., Frey, K. S., Greenberg, M. T., Haynes, N. M., Kessler, R., Schwab-Stone, M. E., & Shriver, T. P. (1997). Promoting social and emotional learning: Guidelines for educators. Alexandria, VA: Association for Supervision and Curriculum Development.

Goldstein, A. P. (1999). *The prepare curriculum: Teaching prosocial competencies* (Rev. ed.). Champaign, IL: Research Press.

Haynie, D. L., Nansel, T., Eitel, P., Crump, A. D., Saylor, K., Yu, K., & Simons-Morton, B. (2001). Bullies, victims, and bully/victims: Distinct groups of at-risk youth. *Journal of Early Adolescence, 2,* 29-49.

Henning-Stout, M., James, S., & Macintosh, S. (2000). Reducing harassment of lesbian, gay, bisexual, transgender, and questioning youth in schools. *School Psychology Review, 29,* 180-192.

Human Rights Watch. (2001). *Hatred in the hallways.* New York: Author.

Knoff, H. M., & Batsche, G. M. (1995). Project ACHIEVE: Analyzing a school reform process for at-risk and underachieving students. *School Psychology Review, 24*(4), 579-603.

Kopels, S., & Dupper, D. R. (1999). School-based peer sexual harassment. *Child Welfare, 78*(4), 435-460.

Layman, N. S. (1994). *Sexual harassment in American secondary schools.* Dallas, TX: Contemporary Research Press.

Lee, V. E., Croninger, R. G., Linn, E., & Chen, X. (1996). The culture of sexual harassment in secondary schools. *American Educational Research Journal, 33,* 383-417.

Lehr, C. A. & Christenson, S. L. (2002). Best practices in promoting a positive school climate. In A. Thomas & J. Grimes (Eds.), *Best practices in school psychology IV–Volume 2* (pp. 929-947). Bethesda, MD: National Association of School Psychologists.

Levy, A. C. & Paludi, M. A. (2002). *Workplace sexual harassment* (2nd ed.). Upper Saddle River, NJ: Prentice Hall.

Minnesota Department of Education. (1993). *Girls and boys getting along. Sexual harassment prevention in the elementary grades.* St. Paul, MN: Author.

Minnesota Department of Education. (1993). *Sexual harassment to teenagers: It's not fun/it's illegal.* St. Paul, MN. Department of Education: Author.

Paludi, M. A. (1997). Sexual harassment in schools. In W. O'Donohue (Ed.), *Sexual harassment: Theory, research, and treatment* (pp. 225-240). Needham Heights, MA: Allyn and Bacon, Inc.

Paludi, M. A., & Barickman, R. B. (1998). *Sexual harassment, work, and education: A resource manual for prevention*. Albany, NY: State University of New York Press.

Raffaele Mendez, L. M., Knoff, H. M., & Ferron, J. (2002). School demographic variables and out-of-school suspension rates: A quantitative and qualitative analysis of a large, ethnically diverse school district. *Psychology in the Schools, 30(3)*, 259-277.

Shoop, R. J., & Edwards, D. L. (1994). *How to stop sexual harassment in our schools: A handbook and curriculum guide for administrators and teachers*. Boston: Allyn & Bacon.

Shoop, R. J., & Hayhow, J. W. (1994). *Sexual harassment in our schools: What parents and teachers need to know to spot it and stop it*. Needham Heights, MA 02194.

Stein, N. (1993). Breaking through casual attitudes on sexual harassment. *Education Digest, 58(9)*, 7-10.

Stein, N. (1995). Sexual harassment in school: The public performance of gendered violence. *Harvard Educational Review, 65(2)*, 145-162.

Stein, N. (1999). *Classrooms & courtrooms: Facing sexual harassment in K-12 schools*. New York: Teachers College Press.

Stein, N., & Sjostrom, L. (1994). *Flirting or hurting? A teachers' guide on student-to-student sexual harassment in schools (grades 6-12)*. Washington, DC: National Education Association.

Stone, C. B. (2000). Advocacy for sexual harassment victims: Legal support and ethical aspects. *Professional School Counseling, 4*, 23-30.

Strauss, S. (1988). Sexual harassment in the school: Legal implications for principals. *National Association of Secondary School Principals Bulletin, 72(506)*, 93-97.

United States Department of Education, Office for Civil Rights and National Association of Attorneys General. (1999). *Protecting students from harassment and hate crime: A guide for schools*. Washington, DC: U.S. Department of Education: Author. Retrieved March 1, 2002, from http://www.ed.gov/pubs/Harassment/

United States Department of Education, Office for Civil Rights. (2001). *Sexual harassment policy guidance: Harassment of students by school employees, other students, or third parties*. Washington, DC: U.S. Department of Education: Author. Retrieved January 14, 2002, from http://www.ed.gov/office/OCR/shguide/index.html

United States Department of Education, Office for Civil Rights. (2002). *Sexual harassment: It's not academic*. [Pamphlet]. Washington, DC: U.S. Department of Education: Author. Retrieved January 14, 2002, from http://www.ed.gov/office/OCR/docs/ocrshpam.html

Webb, L. D., Hunnicutt, K. H., & Metha, A. (1997). What schools can do to combat student-to-student sexual harassment. *National Association of Secondary School Principals Bulletin, 81(585)*, 72-79.

Witt, J. C. (1986). Teachers' resistance to the use of school-based interventions. *Journal of School Psychology, 24*, 37-44.

Dynamics of Peer Victimization in Early Adolescence: Results from a Four-Year Longitudinal Study

Jennifer J. Paul
Antonius H. N. Cillessen

University of Connecticut

SUMMARY. This study addressed the stability of victimization across four consecutive years from Grades 4 to 7, and the concurrent correlates, short-term consequences, and predictors of victimization in early adolescence. Participants were 600 students (49% girls) enrolled in 10 elementary schools in Grades 4-5 and 2 middle schools in Grades 6-7 in an ethnically diverse school system. Data collection included peer nominations, self-reports, and teacher reports in each year. Victimization was highly stable across all years, including the transition from elementary to

---

Address correspondence to: Antonius H. N. Cillessen, Department of Psychology, University of Connecticut, 406 Babbidge Road, Storrs, CT 06269-1020 (E-mail: antonius.cillessen@uconn.edu).

This research was supported by a University of Connecticut Research Foundation faculty grant awarded to the second author. The authors are grateful to the students and teachers who participated in the study and wish to acknowledge the assistance provided by the school administrators. Parts of this research were presented at the annual meeting of the American Psychological Association, Washington, DC, August, 2000.

[Haworth co-indexing entry note]: "Dynamics of Peer Victimization in Early Adolescence: Results from a Four-Year Longitudinal Study." Paul, Jennifer J., and Antonius H. N. Cillessen. Co-published simultaneously in *Journal of Applied School Psychology* (The Haworth Press, Inc.) Vol. 19, No. 2, 2003, pp. 25-43; and: *Bullying, Peer Harassment, and Victimization in the Schools: The Next Generation of Prevention* (ed: Maurice J. Elias, and Joseph E. Zins) The Haworth Press, Inc., 2003, pp. 25-43. Single or multiple copies of this article are available for a fee from The Haworth Document Delivery Service [1-800-HAWORTH, 9:00 a.m. - 5:00 p.m. (EST). E-mail address: docdelivery@haworthpress.com].

10.1300/J008v19n02_03

middle school. Both concurrent and short-term consequences showed that victimized 6th graders, especially girls, experienced significantly greater maladaptive outcomes than their nonvictim counterparts. For both genders, risk factors for adolescent victimization included externalizing and internalizing behaviors, while protective factors included academic and peer sociability elements. Implications for prevention and intervention are discussed. *[Article copies available for a fee from The Haworth Document Delivery Service: 1-800-HAWORTH. E-mail address: <docdelivery@haworthpress.com> Website: <http://www.HaworthPress.com> © 2003 by The Haworth Press, Inc. All rights reserved.]*

KEYWORDS. Victimization, stability, risk factors, adjustment, gender differences

Early adolescence is a crucial period of development due to the many biological, cognitive, and social changes that occur during this time. Peer relationships and interactions during the middle school years greatly influence differentiation and individuation of self-concepts. It is during early adolescence that an extremely fragile sense of self begins to unfold. Adolescents in this stage of development are able to recognize contradictions in their self-concepts and in how they conceptualize others, but they are not yet able to explain or reconcile these contradictions (Harter, 1998). Experiences during this time of social development will shape eventual identity formation in later adolescence and early adulthood.

Considering the impact of peer relations on normative social development during early adolescence, it follows that studying peer harassment or victimization that occurs during this time is critical. Peer relations researchers have considered various forms of peer harassment, including being a victim of physical, direct verbal, and indirect verbal aggression (Underwood, Galen, & Paquette, 2001). Although researchers in this area of study have often explored victimization in elementary school samples (e.g., Crick & Bigbee, 1998; Hodges, Boivin, Vitaro, & Bukowski, 1999; Kochenderfer-Ladd & Wardrop, 2001), less is known about this phenomenon in adolescence. One reason for this is that victimization is often assessed using peer nominations, and sociometric methods had not been used very often in early adolescent groups until recently. It is, however, crucial to explore victimization further in the early adolescent years because the experience of victimization may be especially detrimental at this time of identity formation and development of peer interactions and relationships.

STABILITY OF VICTIMIZATION

The stability of physically aggressive behavior is a well-documented finding (Coie & Dodge, 1998). Individual differences in aggression are stable over time and consistent across changes in peer group composition. Less is known, however, about the stability of being the target of peer aggression or victimization. Understanding the stability of victimization is crucial because victimization is a serious problem for students who are frequently its targets.

Most research on the stability of victimization has focused on frequency rather than chronicity (Boulton & Smith, 1994; Boulton & Underwood, 1992). Kochenderfer-Ladd and Wardrop (2001) examined physical, verbal, indirect verbal, and general victimization, and suggested that chronic victimization is not as common as might be expected based on frequency studies. This finding may be due in part to their focus on children in early elementary school only. Victimization may become more stable over the course of development and especially in early adolescence (Hodges & Perry, 1999). The stability of victimization needs to be considered not only across time, but also across contexts, keeping in mind potential changes in peer group composition. In this respect, the change from elementary to middle school, especially when it results in a new peer group, is an important developmental transition. If victimization is highly stable across time and contexts, it is critical to intervene at the earliest sign of victimization rather than believing that victimization is an experience that will pass.

Correlates and Consequences of Victimization

Research has shown that the experience of victimization is tied to emotional distress such as loneliness, anxiety, and depression (see, for a review, Kochenderfer-Ladd & Ladd, 2001) and to maladjustment as reflected in poor school achievement, self-confidence, self-esteem, and prosocial skills (Kochenderfer & Ladd, 1996; Perry, Perry, & Kennedy, 1992). These correlates of victimization have been explored in not only North American children, but also children in other cultures. For children between 9 and 12 years old in Greece (Andreou, 2001), in China (Schwartz, Chang, & Farver, 2001), and Turkish children living in The Netherlands (Verkuyten & Thijs, 2001), the experience of victimization has been found to be negatively correlated with self-worth and academic functioning, and positively correlated with behavior problems. Researchers in England (Mynard, Joseph, & Alexander, 2000) and South Australia (Rigby, 2000) studied 12- to 16-year-old adolescents and found victimization to be correlated with increased psychological distress (e.g., anxiety, depression) and diminished self-worth. Since many of the present studies of the concurrent correlates of victimization rely solely on self-report, however, researchers must continue to explore these by building upon the few studies that have used a multi-informant approach (e.g., Boivin, Hymel, & Hodges, 2001; Schwartz et al., 2001).

While it is clear that social maladjustment occurs concurrently with the experience of victimization, a number of studies have suggested that many of the concurrent correlates of victimization are also short-term consequences of victimization. For example, Hodges et al. (1999) found that victimized children without a mutual best friend experience both internalizing and externalizing problems one year later. In addition, increased truancy and a decline in academic performance in the spring of one academic year have been identified as short-term consequences of being victimized the previous fall (Kochenderfer & Ladd, 1996).

Furthermore, the experience of victimization at the hands of peers predicts retaliatory violence by the victims, who may imitate the aggression to which they have been chronically subjected. Various studies have demonstrated an association between victimization and aggression; between 5% and 10% of children who are the victims of peer aggression are themselves aggressive towards others (Olweus, 1978; Pellegrini, Bartini, & Brooks, 1999; Perry et al., 1992; Schwartz, Dodge, Pettit, & Bates, 1997). These children often become involved in emotionally charged conflicts that they tend to mismanage (Perry et al., 1992). Reports in the media of teenagers who have been involved in school shootings have suggested that these students often had a history of peer victimization before they became violent themselves. Isaacs, Card, and Hodges (2000) shed further light on this anecdotal information by showing that early adolescent boys (girls report never carrying weapons) who score high on both victimization and aggression are the most likely to carry weapons to middle school. Thus, victimization may play an important role in the occurrence of violence in school.

Predictors of Victimization

In addition to examining the concurrent behavioral and sociocognitive correlates and short-term consequences, the predictors of victimization are equally important. Elementary school students have been the focus of most of the current studies on the predictors of victimization. These studies have suggested that low self-perceived social competence, poor peer relations, internalizing and externalizing problems, and physical weakness may be predictors of elementary school victimization (see, for a review, Perry, Hodges, & Egan, 2001).

Hodges and Perry (1999) conducted one of the few studies that included older children when they examined the antecedents of victimization in third through seventh graders across a one-year interval. They found that internalizing problems, physical weakness, and peer rejection each contributed to later victimization. However, relatively little is known about the antecedents of victimization over longer intervals and into adolescence. This information is important from an early intervention perspective. Knowledge of the early predictors helps school administrators to identify students who are most likely to become victims later and to plan interventions accordingly. Intervention should address not only victimization in a proactive manner, but bullying as well. Teaching and encouraging children to embrace and value diversity, acquire team-building skills, and develop effective anger management and conflict resolution strategies at an early age are key in this effort.

Current Study

Given these considerations, the goal of the current study was to contribute to what is known about the role of victimization in adolescent development, and identify potential points of prevention and intervention by examining in detail the correlates, outcomes, and predictors of victimization in early adolescence. General victimization, including physical, direct verbal, and indirect verbal forms, was examined. The specific research hypotheses were: (1) victimization is expected to be stable across four consecutive school years (Grades 4-7), including the transition from elementary to middle school; (2) victimization is expected to be related to concurrent measures of social and academic functioning at school in early adolescence (Grade 6); (3) victimization is expected to be negatively related to short-term adjustment outcomes in early adolescence (Grade 7); (4) both internalizing withdrawal behaviors and externalizing disruptive behaviors in elementary school (Grades 4-5) are expected to be predictors of early adolescent victimization, while self-efficacy and positive peer relationships are expected to protect against later victimization; and (5) previous research has indicated that the dynamics of peer victimization may differ for boys and girls, but the reported differences are highly variable from study to study making it difficult to hypothesize specific differences. Therefore, the examination of gender differences within the dynamics of peer victimization is treated as exploratory.

METHOD

Participants and Design

Data collection took place in the spring of four consecutive school years as students from one cohort were followed longitudinally from Grade 4 to Grade 7. In each year, all students were invited to participate in the study. The participation rate was 95% or higher in each year, resulting in sample sizes of 658, 638, 600, and 600, for Grades 4-7, respectively. In Grades 4 and 5, participants were enrolled in 28 classrooms of 10 elementary schools. In Grades 6 and 7, they converged into two middle schools. No formal bullying interventions were taking place at any of these schools at the time of the study. About 50% of the students in each year were girls. The ethnic composition of the sample at the beginning of the study (Grade 4) was 77% White, 14% Black, 8% Latino, and 1% of other origin. The data collection in each year included a peer sociometric measure as well as self- and teacher-report measures; these are discussed below.

Peer Sociometric Measures

Victimization was assessed in each year using unlimited peer nominations with grade as the reference group, allowing same-sex and other-sex choices. Confidentiality was discussed preceding the peer nominations. Students were instructed to work by themselves and respect each other's privacy, and researchers monitored the data collection to ensure that students complied with these guidelines. Information about individual students was not accessible to teachers or school administrators.

In each grade, a general victimization question was used ("Name the people in your grade who get picked on and teased by other kids"). In Grades 6 and 7, two additional questions were used, one for physical victimization ("Name the people who get hit, pushed, or kicked by others") and one for relational victimization ("Name the people who have lies, rumors, or mean things said about them"). In each year, nominations received were counted and standardized within school by computing z-scores. This method is consistent with the usual procedures for processing peer nomination data (cf. Cillessen & Bellmore, 1999). In Grades 4 and 5, each student's victimization score was the standardized number of general victimization nominations received. In Grades 6 and 7, the standard scores for the three victimization items were highly correlated (all r's > .75). Therefore, they were averaged to one victimization composite score in each year. In order to identify victimization status in Grade 6, students with a z-score larger than 1 for general, physical, or relational victimization were identified as victims ($n = 68$; 46 boys, 22 girls). The remaining sixth graders ($n = 531$; 260 boys, 271 girls) formed the nonvictimized comparison group.

Teacher Ratings

As part of the larger study, teachers rated students on a variety of constructs each year. Teachers completed the teacher report forms while students completed the peer nomination and self-report forms. Of interest for the present study were teacher ratings of disruptive conduct, school competence, and peer sociability. Items for each construct were selected from existing instruments that were age-appropriate for each grade and, therefore, varied somewhat from year to year. To place all resulting scores on a comparable metric scale, scores were standardized to z-scores in each year.

In Grades 4 and 5, three items were available for each construct from the teacher form of the Child Rating Scale (T-CRS; Hightower, Work, Cowen, Lotyczewski, Spinell, Guare, & Rohrbeck, 1986), except that one item was available for peer sociability in Grade 4. All items were rated on a 9-point scale to indicate how much they described a student (1 = not at all, 9 = very much). Internal consistencies (Cronbach's α) were .83 and .88 (disruptive conduct) and .88 and .92 (school competence) in Grades 4 and 5, respectively, and .94 for sociability (Grade 5).

In Grades 6 and 7, six items were available to measure disruptive conduct from the teacher form of the Child Behavior Checklist (CBCL; Achenbach, 1991a). Four items from the Multidimensional Self-concept Scale (MSCS; Bracken, 1992) were available to measure school competence and peer sociability. All items were rated on a 7-point scale indicating how much they were true for each student (1 = not at all, 7 = very much). Internal consistencies (Cronbach's α) were .90 and .91 (disruptive conduct), .88 and .87 (school competence), and .92 and .91 (peer sociability) in Grades 6 and 7, respectively.

Self-Report Measures

Students rated themselves in each year on six constructs within the larger longitudinal study that were of interest for the purpose of the present study: internalizing problems (loneliness or depression), disruptive conduct, anxiety/withdrawal, peer sociability, social self-efficacy, and academic self-efficacy. In addition, because self- and other-awareness become important in adolescence, meta-perceptions of victimization, cooperation, aggression, and withdrawal were also assessed in middle school. Items for each construct were selected from existing instruments that were age-appropriate for each age group and, therefore, varied somewhat from year to year. To correct for variation in the metrics of ratings between years, scale scores in each year were standardized to z-scores. The measures selected for the present study are described below.

Internalizing problems. In Grades 4 and 5, loneliness was assessed with the 24-item Loneliness and Social Dissatisfaction Inventory (Asher & Wheeler, 1985) ($\alpha = .88$ and .91 in Grades 4 and 5, respectively). In Grade 6, depression was assessed with the 26-item Child Depression Inventory (CDI; Kovacs, 1992; $\alpha = .77$). In Grade 7, depression was assessed with the 12-item Beck Depression Inventory (BDI; Beck, Steer, & Garbin, 1988; $\alpha = .85$).

Behavior ratings. In Grades 4 and 5, participants rated their disruptive conduct, anxiety/withdrawal, and peer sociability with six items (Grade 4) or four items (Grade 5) per construct selected from the child form of the Child Rating Scale (CRS; Hightower, Cowen, Spinell, Lotyczewski, Guare, Rohrbeck, & Brown, 1987). Items were rated on a 5-point scale indicating how well they described the student (1 = not at all true, 5 = always true). Internal consistencies were .84 and .79 (disruptive conduct), .81 and .67 (anxious-withdrawn), and .82 and .81 (peer sociability) in Grades 4 and 5, respectively.

In Grades 6 and 7, participants rated their disruptive conduct on 12 items selected from the child form of the CBCL (Achenbach, 1991b). Twelve items derived from the MSCS (Bracken, 1992) were available for school competence and peer sociability. All items were rated on a 7-point scale indicating how much they were true for a student (1 = not at all, 7 = always). Internal consistencies were .83 and .86 (disruptive conduct), .87 and .91 (anxious-withdrawn), and .66 and .84 (peer sociability) in Grades 6 and 7, respectively.

Self-efficacy. Social and academic self-efficacy were measured in Grades 5, 6, and 7 with items from the Student Self-concept Scale (SSCS; Gresham, Elliot, & Evans-Fernandez, 1993). These constructs were not assessed in Grade 4. Twenty items measuring social self-efficacy were available in Grades 5 and 7 ($\alpha = .89$ and .93), and 11 items in Grade 6 ($\alpha = .89$). Academic self-efficacy was measured with 18 items in Grades 5 and 7 ($\alpha = .89$ and .92) and with 9 items in Grade 6 ($\alpha = .91$). Students rated all items on a 5-point scale (Grade 5) or 7-point scale (Grades 6 and 7), indicating how confident they were in their ability to engage in the behavior described by each item (1 = not at all confident, 5 or 7 = very confident). Scale scores were averaged across items and standardized to z-scores to make them comparable between measures and years.

Meta-perceptions. Adolescents' beliefs about how others saw them were assessed in Grades 6 and 7 for victimization ("How many people in your grade think that you get picked on and teased by other kids?"), prosocial behavior ("How many people in your grade think that you cooperate, share, or help others?"), aggression ("How many people in your grade think that you start fights, say mean things, or tease others?"), and social withdrawal ("How many people in your grade think that you are hard to get to know because you stay by yourself a lot?"). Students rated each item on a 7-point scale (1 = almost no one, 7 = almost everyone).

RESULTS

Stability of Victimization

First, correlations were computed between the continuous peer-nomination-based victimization scores for Grades 4 through 7. All correlations were significant ($p < .05$). The 1-year stability of victimization was about equally high in elementary school (.70) and in middle school (.68). Despite the change in social context and peer group, the 1-year stability of victimization across the transition from elementary to middle school was high as well (.62). The 2-year stabilities that included the school transition were almost as high (.60 and .58). The stability of victimization from Grades 4 to 7 was lower (.44), but still substantial.

Second, stability of victimization was examined categorically. Consistent with previous approaches, students with a victimization z-score larger than +1 in each year were classified as victims. Of the students who were victims in Grade 4, 65% were also victims in Grade 5, 49% in Grade 6, and 34% in Grade 7. Of the Grade 5 victims, 42% and 43% were also victims in Grades 6 and 7, respectively. Finally, 48% of the victims in Grade 6 were also victims in Grade 7.

Both the continuous and categorical approaches indicated significant stability of victimization across the four years of the study. The continuous and categorical stabilities for boys and girls separately were identical to each other and to the results for the total sample.

Concurrent Correlates of Adolescent Victimization

A 2 (Grade 6 Victimization Status; Victim vs. Nonvictim) × 2 (Gender) ANOVA was conducted on the Grade 6 teacher- and self-report measures. Multiple ANOVAs were run following the statistical argumentation of Huberty and Morris (1989). A significant effect of victimization was found for teacher ratings of disruptive behavior, $F(1, 446) = 13.49$, school competence, $F(1, 445) = 15.27$, and peer sociability, $F(1, 446) = 9.14$, and for self-ratings of disruptive behavior, $F(1, 464) = 15.00$, withdrawal, $F(1, 464) = 5.48$, peer sociability, $F(1, 464) = 9.39$, perceived aggression, $F(1, 456) = 18.20$, perceived victimization, $F(1, 450) = 16.55$, all p's $< .003$, and academic self-efficacy, $F(1, 431) = 4.01$, $p = .046$. As can be seen in Table 1, victims scored higher than nonvictims on disruptive behavior (teacher and self), withdrawal, and perceived aggression and victimization. Victims scored lower than nonvictims on school competence, peer sociability (teacher and self), and academic self-efficacy.

Several significant effects of gender were found. Teachers rated girls (M = .19, SD = .97) higher than boys (M = $-.18$, SD = .99) on peer sociability, $F(1, 446) = 7.04$, $p = .008$. They also rated girls (M = .16, SD = .91) higher than boys (M = $-.16$, SD = 1.06) on school competence, $F(1, 445) = 5.39$, $p = .021$. On self-reports of disruptive behavior, boys (M = .15, SD = 1.06) scored higher than girls (M = $-.16$, SD = .90), $F(1, 464) = 4.19$, $p = .041$. On self-reports of anxiety-withdrawal, girls (M = .13, SD = .98) scored higher than boys (M = $-.13$, SD = 1.00), $F(1, 464) = 4.82$, $p = .029$. On perceived prosocial behavior, girls (M = .22, SD = .91) also scored higher than boys (M = $-.21$, SD = 1.04) did, $F(1, 457) = 4.42$, $p = .036$.

The effect of victimization on academic self-efficacy was qualified by an interaction with gender, $F(1, 431) = 5.97$, $p = .015$. Victimization influenced academic self-efficacy for girls only, $F(1, 217) = 11.01$, $p < .001$. Victimized girls (M = $-.52$, SD = 1.35) had lower academic self-efficacy expectations than nonvictimized girls (M = .20, SD = .80) did. Victimized boys (M = $-.08$, SD = 1.09) did not differ from other boys (M = $-.15$, SD = 1.10).

To further examine the concurrent associations of victimization, a stepwise regression analysis was conducted in which the continuous victimization score in Grade 6 was regressed on the concurrent teacher- and self-report measures. The final model included six predictors explaining 22% of the variance in victimization, $F(6, 316) = 15.06$, $p < .001$. Not surprisingly, self-reported disruptive conduct ($\beta = .22$) and perceived victimization ($\beta = .19$) positively predicted victimization, whereas teacher-reported school competence ($\beta = -.30$) and self-reported peer sociability ($\beta = -.14$) negatively predicted victimization.

Interestingly, social self-efficacy was also a positive predictor ($\beta = .21$), and social isolation a negative predictor of victimization ($\beta = -.12$). These effects seem counterintuitive at first, as self-efficacy is typically associated with positive outcome and social isolation with negative outcome. In the context of victimization, however, they make sense when considering that both are related to the frequency with which students expose themselves to peer interaction. Socially self-efficacious students engage themselves frequently in interactions with peers, thereby also increasing the risk that some of these interactions may be met with rebuff. Isolated students limit their interactions, and thereby decrease the risk that some interactions turn out negative. Thus, we predict that these effects are mediated by frequency of interaction, and will disappear when it is controlled for, a hypothesis to be tested in further research.

Short-Term Consequences of Adolescent Victimization

A 2 (Grade 6 Victimization Status) × 2 (Gender) ANCOVA was conducted on each Grade 7 teacher- and self-report measure, using the equivalent Grade 6 measure as a covariate. Thus, we tested whether Grade 6 victims and nonvictims were significantly different from one another one year later in Grade 7, after controlling for their initial differences in Grade 6. Multiple ANCOVAs were run, following the arguments of Huberty und Morris (1989).

A significant effect of Grade 6 victimization was found on Grade 7 teacher-rated peer sociability, $F(1, 363) = 16.72$, $p < .001$, and self-rated disruptive behavior, $F(1, 362) = 5.21$, $p = .023$, anxiety-withdrawal, $F(1, 363) = 5.24$, $p = .023$, peer sociability, $F(1, 362) = 7.45$, $p = .007$, social self-efficacy, $F(1, 324) = 4.00$, $p = .046$, and perceived prosocial behavior, $F(1, 358) = 7.98$, $p = .005$, controlling for these variables in Grade 6. The interpretation of these effects is aided by the adjusted means in Table 1, indicating which group

TABLE 1. Means and Standard Deviations in Grade 6 and Adjusted Means and Standard Errors in Grade 7 for Students Who Were Victims and Nonvictims in Grade 6

| | Grade 6 | | | | Grade 7 | | | |
| | M | | SD | | M_{adj} | | SE | |
	V	NV	V	NV	V	NV	V	NV
Disruptive (T)	*.54*	−.06	1.17	.96	−.04	−.04	.15	.05
School competence (T)	*−.62*	*.07*	1.10	.96	−.04	.06	.17	.05
Peer sociability (T)	*−.50*	*.06*	1.00	.98	*−.57*	*.10*	.16	.05
Disruptive (S)	*.57*	*−.07*	1.08	.97	*.28*	*−.02*	.12	.04
Anxious-withdrawn (S)	*.27*	*−.03*	.99	.10	*.21*	*−.04*	.13	.04
Peer sociability (S)	*−.45*	*.05*	1.15	.97	*−.34*	*.08*	.14	.05
Depression (S)	.19	−.02	.93	1.01	.19	−.06	.14	.05
Social self-efficacy (S)	−.05	.01	1.10	.99	*−.16*	*.14*	.14	.05
Academic self-efficacy (S)	*−.25*	*.03*	1.21	.97	.03	.07	.14	.04
Perceived prosocial (S)	−.12	.01	.98	1.00	*−.38*	*.06*	.15	.05
Perceived aggression (S)	*.60*	*−.07*	1.30	.93	.21	−.08	.15	.05
Perceived withdrawal (S)	.05	−.01	1.00	1.00	.20	−.06	.15	.05
Perceived victimization (S)	*.63*	*−.07*	1.34	.93	.21	.02	.17	.06

Note. V = victim; NV = nonvictim; T = teacher-report; S = self-report. Means (Grade 6) and adjusted means (Grade 7) that are underlined are significantly different between victims and nonvictims.

scored higher and which group scored lower compared to one another. Compared to nonvictims, being a victim in Grade 6 was associated with decreased sociability and social self-efficacy in Grade 7, increased disruptive and anxious-withdrawn behavior, and enhanced beliefs of being viewed negatively by peers (as anxious-withdrawn and not prosocial).

A significant effect of gender was found for self-ratings of depression, $F(1, 357) = 13.67$, anxiety-withdrawal, $F(1, 363) = 15.62$, and perceived prosocial behavior, $F(1, 358) = 6.86$, p's $< .009$. Girls had higher scores than boys for depression ($M_{adj} = .34$ vs. $-.21$, $SE = .11$ vs. $.10$) and anxiety-withdrawal ($M_{adj} = .38$ vs. $-.15$, $SE = .10$ vs. $.09$). Boys were less likely to think that peers saw them as prosocial ($M_{adj} = -.36$ vs. $.05$, $SE = .10$ vs. $.12$).

A significant victim by gender interaction was found for depression, $F(1, 357) = 10.79$, $p = .001$, anxiety-withdrawal, $F(1, 363) = 9.13$, $p = .003$, self-rated disruptive behavior, $F(1, 362) = 11.19$, $p < .001$, peer sociability, $F(1, 362) = 4.67$, $p = .031$, and perceived anxiety-withdrawal, $F(1, 354) = 6.26$, $p = .013$. These interactions reflected that victimized girls stood out from the other groups. As seen in Table 2, victimized girls were more depressed and withdrawn than all other groups, who did not differ from each other. Victimized girls believed that peers saw them as more anxious-withdrawn than did nonvictimized girls, whereas victimized and nonvictimized boys did not differ. Victimized girls rated themselves as more disruptive and less sociable with peers than did nonvictimized girls and boys. Among nonvictims, boys were more disruptive than girls; among victims, girls were more disruptive than boys.

TABLE 2. Adjusted Means and Standard Errors for Self-Ratings in Grade 7 for Victimized and Nonvictimized Girls and Boys

	M_{adj}				SE			
	Girls		Boys		Girls		Boys	
	V	NV	V	NV	V	NV	V	NV
Depression	$.70_a$	$-.03_b$	$-.32_b$	$-.09_b$	.21	.07	.18	.07
Anxious-withdrawn	$.74_a$	$.03_b$	$-.20_b$	$-.10_b$	.20	.06	.17	.06
Perceived withdrawal	$.51_a$	$-.14_b$	$-.12_b$	$.01_b$	.23	.07	.19	.07
Peer sociability	$-.61_a$	$.13_b$	$-.07_{ab}$	$.02_b$	.22	.07	.19	.07
Disruptive	$.58_a$	$-.15_b$	$-.03_{bc}$	$.11_c$	.19	.06	.16	.06

Note. V = victim; NV = nonvictim. Means in the same row that do not share subscripts differ at $p < .05$ in a post-hoc comparison test.

To further examine the effect of victimization on later adjustment, a series of hierarchical regressions was run in which each Grade 7 measure was predicted from its equivalent Grade 6 measure in Step 1, after which the incremental effect of Grade 6 victimization (continuous score) was tested in Step 2. Being victimized in Grade 6 significantly and incrementally predicted lower teacher ratings of peer sociability ($\beta = -.21$), and self-ratings reflecting more disruptive conduct ($\beta = .11$), less social self-efficacy ($\beta = -.11$), and beliefs of being seen more negatively by peers as less prosocial ($\beta = -.17$), more aggressive ($\beta = .14$), and more socially isolated ($\beta = .14$).

Risk and Protective Factors of Adolescent Victimization

To examine the effects of potential risk and protective factors on adolescent victimization, composite scores were computed for nine measures assessed in elementary school by averaging them across the Grade 4 and 5 assessments (except for efficacy measures, which were only assessed in Grade 5). Loneliness, anxiety, and disruptive behavior (teachers and self) were considered risk factors of adolescent victimization. School competence, social and academic self-efficacy, and peer sociability (teachers and self) were considered protective factors. All nine factors were entered into a discriminant analysis to examine their ability to determine victim status in Grade 6, following the transition to middle school. The discriminant analysis was run twice, once for boys and once for girls.

A significant linear discriminant function was found for girls, $F(9, 229) = 2.11$, $p = .029$, correctly classifying 68% of Grade 6 victims, and 72% of nonvictims. Consistent with the expectations, function coefficients for the classification of victim status were positive for the risk factors loneliness (.19, ns.), anxiety-withdrawal (.40, $p = .071$), disruptive behavior-self (.54, $p = .014$), and disruptive behavior-teacher (.41, $p = .060$), and negative for the protective factors social self-efficacy ($-.16$, ns.), academic self-efficacy ($-.55$, $p = .013$), peer sociability-self ($-.52, p = .017$), peer sociability-teacher ($-.42, p = .056$), and school competence ($-.43, p = .052$). Thus, disruptive behavior in elementary school was the strongest risk factor for later victimization for girls, followed by anxious-withdrawn behavior. Academic self-efficacy, school competence, and peer sociability were the strongest protective factors against victimization for girls.

A significant linear discriminant function was also found for boys, $F(9, 243) = 2.08$, $p = .032$, correctly classifying 60% of Grade 6 victims, and 70% of nonvictims. Again, consistent with the expectations, function coefficients for the classification of victim status were positive for the risk factors loneliness (.30, $p = .049$), anxiety-withdrawal (.11, ns.), disruptive behavior-self (.34, $p = .027$), and disruptive behavior-teacher (.42, $p = .006$), and negative for the protective factors social self-efficacy (−.19, ns.), academic self-efficacy (−.26, $p = .091$), peer sociability-self (−.37, $p = .015$), peer sociability-teacher (−.57, $p = .001$), and school competence (−.48, $p = .001$). Thus, disruptive behavior in elementary school was the strongest risk factor for later victimization for boys, followed by loneliness. School competence and peer sociability were the strongest protective factors for boys.

DISCUSSION

The goal of this study was to examine the dynamics of peer victimization in a large sample of students as they were followed from elementary school across the transition to middle school. The stability, concurrent correlates, short-term consequences, and predictors of victimization in early adolescence were examined.

The stability of victimization was high across all years of the study. The stability of aggression is often reported to be in the .50-.60 range (see Coie & Dodge, 1998). Remarkably, the stability of victimization in the current study exceeded these estimates. Thus, peer victimization is a highly stable phenomenon across the middle childhood and early adolescent years. We found correlations exceeding .70 across consecutive years, even when this included an important change in social context (and corresponding composition of the peer group). A correlation of .70 translates into a proportion of shared variance of about 50% between consecutive measurement points, indicating that change also occurred in the midst of stability. On the other hand, the .70 stability coefficients are among the highest found for any construct in the social development literature (stabilities of aggression and social preference average around .60), and thus should be taken very seriously. The proportion of stable victims ranged from about two-thirds across the shortest interval (one year) to one-third across the longest interval (four years).

The concurrent correlates of victimization in our current sample corroborate and extend what has been found in previous research. As before, victimized adolescents are characterized by a number of psychosocial adjustment problems that include high levels of internalizing and externalizing behaviors, and low academic expectations (about themselves) and competencies (as reported by their teachers). It should be noted that low academic self-efficacy expectations were particularly characteristic of victimized girls, much more so than of boys and nonvictimized girls. This may be related to some of the other unique characteristics of girls who are victims of peer aggression that are detailed below.

Beyond the concurrent correlates of victimization, a question of great importance is that of causality. Does victimization by peers lead to the maladjustment problems described, or do underlying maladjustment problems predispose a child or adolescent to become an easy target for others? Disentangling causality is complex given the quasi-experimental nature of the majority of research in this field, yet is becoming increasingly possible with advanced statistical methods. The current study made a contribution to this issue by examining whether victimization is associated with later behavior problems when controlling for earlier levels of the outcome variables. In this respect, our study demonstrated a number of important findings strongly suggestive of an effect of victimization on negative outcomes.

The negative short-term consequences of victimization in early adolescence were found for girls, but not for boys. Victimized girls had higher levels of depression, anxiety, negative social self-perceptions, as well as self-reported disruptive behavior after one year than any other group. The question of importance is why this finding is so pronounced for early adolescent girls. Several explanations are possible. One is that girls are generally more accurate social perceivers and more sensitive to rejection than are boys (see, e.g., Cillessen & Bellmore, 1999). In addition, the forms of victimization among adolescent girls are more likely to be socially rather than physically aggressive in nature (Galen & Underwood, 1999). Combining their heightened awareness of social processes with the relational nature of the aggression may explain why victimization is associated with such negative outcomes for girls, particularly in the internalizing domain.

Our results also shed light on the elementary school variables that can be considered risk and protective factors of victimization in adolescence. For both girls and boys, the protective factors had a social and an academic component. For both genders, peer sociability was a protective factor against adolescent victimization. This effect may be direct or indirect. Directly, being more socially skilled enables adolescents to deal more effectively with the social pressures of the peer system. Indirectly, more sociable students are more likely to have friends or belong to social groups that may serve as a buffer against victimization. Teacher ratings of school competence and academic self-efficacy were associated with reduced risk of victimization for both genders. Academic achievement and confidence may be related to a more general sense of self-confidence in the school environment that may make students less vulnerable to peer harassment.

Early risk factors were also quite similar for girls and boys, and included both an externalizing and an internalizing component. For both genders, disruptive behavior in elementary school was associated with victim status in middle school. Disruptive behavior may be a risk factor because it is associated with poor behavioral and emotional regulation, making children easy to antagonize. Also, the disregulated reactions of these children are reinforcing for peers who victimize them. It is also possible that students may turn to disruptive behavior as a reaction to being victimized. Thus, disruptive behavior may become both a cause and consequence within the dynamics of victimization. The same may hold true for the internalizing risk factors, specifically, anxious-withdrawn behavior for girls and loneliness for boys. Being anxious or withdrawn and lacking a peer support network make a child defenseless, vulnerable, and an easy target for bullying. Again, these internalizing behaviors may be not only risk factors for future victimization, but also a result of previous victimization, thus placing the child in a vicious cycle of victimization experiences from which it is difficult to escape.

Strengths and Limitations

A number of strengths and limitations of the current study warrant mention. Strengths of the current study are the large sample size and the ability to make gender comparisons. Also, the longitudinal nature of the research design, spanning an extended period of time, enabled us to examine predictors as well as consequences in the context of a single study. Finally, by using peer nominations, self-report measures, and teacher reports, the current study followed a multi-informant approach that is important for work in this area.

Limitations of the current study need to be examined as well. One limitation is that, although often developmentally appropriate, the change in number of items used to measure certain constructs over the course of the study may hinder some comparisons. Also, because the study was limited to one cohort, it cannot speak to potential differences across cohorts. Finally, there is a limitation in the causal interpretation of the data due to potential mediating and moderating factors (e.g., family influences) that are unknown. Further examination of mediating and moderating factors is an important direction for future research.

Implications for Research and Intervention

From a prevention standpoint, our data demonstrated that there are a number of behaviors of children in elementary school that function as risk and protective factors of later victimization. Risk factors included both internalizing and externalizing behaviors. Elementary school children who experience problems in these domains would be selected for intervention efforts aimed at alleviating these problems. The fact that these behaviors are also related to later victimization makes early intervention even more important. On the positive side, protective factors for victimization included school competence and peer sociability. Again, while the strengthening of academic and social skills are obviously of primary importance in and of themselves, the fact that these skills are also protective factors for later victimization contributes further to the importance of their pursuit. Unfortunately, high levels of risk factors tend to co-occur with low levels of protective factors. Children with externalizing or internalizing problems tend also to score low on peer sociability and academic achievement. Thus, children who demonstrate a profile of negative scores across all four of these domains should be considered as particularly at risk for later problems in relationships with peers.

From an intervention perspective, our data clearly indicate and confirm the negative social ramifications of victimization. Interventionists will need to take into consideration and target the internalizing problems of victimized adolescents. Efforts at reducing these problems will be ineffective if the processes of bullying in the peer group are allowed to continue and not addressed directly as well. Furthermore, it seems likely that labeling the victim as a "problem student" or "someone who needs help" will not contribute to eliminating the targeting of this person by peers in her or his daily life in school. Thus, intervention needs to be systemic, focusing on the peer system as a whole, rather than only examining the individual. It may be possible to address bullying and victimization directly through student initiatives and peer-run groups or clubs (see Peterson & Rigby, 1999). Incorporating team-building and conflict-management skill development into these groups or clubs may serve to improve social skills and, in turn, impede the cycle of bullying and victimization.

REFERENCES

Achenbach, T. M. (1991a). *Manual for the Teacher's Report Form and 1991 Profile.* Burlington, VT: University of Vermont Department of Psychiatry.
Achenbach, T. M. (1991b). *Manual for the Youth Self-Report and 1991 Profile.* Burlington, VT: University of Vermont Department of Psychiatry.
Andreou, E. (2001). Bully/victim problems and their association with coping behaviour in conflictual peer interactions among school-age children. *Educational Psychology, 21*, 59-66.
Asher, S. R., & Wheeler, V. A. (1985). Children's loneliness: A comparison of rejected and neglected peer status. *Journal of Consulting and Clinical Psychology, 53*, 500-505.
Beck, A. T., Steer, R. A., & Garbin, M. (1988). Psychometric properties of the Beck Depression Inventory: Twenty-five years of evaluation. *Clinical Psychology Review, 8*, 77-100.

Boivin, M., Hymel, S., & Hodges, E. V. E. (2001). Toward a process view of peer rejection and harassment. In J. Juvonen & S. Graham (Eds.), *Peer harassment in school: The plight of the vulnerable and victimized* (pp. 265-289). New York: Guilford Press.

Boulton, M. J., & Smith, P. K. (1994). Bully/victim problems in middle-school children: Stability, self-perceived competence, peer perceptions, and peer acceptance. *British Journal of Developmental Psychology, 12*, 315-329.

Boulton, M. J., & Underwood, K. (1992). Bully/victim problems among middle school children. *British Journal of Educational Psychology, 62*, 73-87.

Bracken, B. A. (1992). *The Multidimensional Self-concept Scale.* Austin, TX: PRO-ED.

Cillessen, A. H. N., & Bellmore, A. D. (1999). Accuracy of social self-perceptions and peer competence in middle childhood. *Merrill-Palmer Quarterly, 45*, 650-676.

Coie, J. D., & Dodge, K. A. (1998). Aggression and antisocial behavior. In W. Damon (Series Ed.) & N. Eisenberg (Vol. Ed.), *Handbook of child psychology: Vol. 3. Social, emotional, and personality development* (5th ed., pp. 779-862). New York: Wiley.

Crick, N. R., & Bigbee, M. A. (1998). Relational and overt forms of peer victimization: A multi-informant approach. *Journal of Consulting and Clinical Psychology, 66*, 237-347.

Egan, S. K., & Perry, D. G. (1998). Does low self-regard invite victimization? *Developmental Psychology, 34*, 299-309.

Galen, B. R., & Underwood, M. K. (1997). A developmental investigation of social aggression among children. *Developmental Psychology, 33*, 589-600.

Gresham, S. M., Elliot, S. N., & Evans-Fernandez, S. E. (1993). *Student Self-concept Scale.* Circle Pines, MN: American Guidance Service, Inc.

Harter, S. (1998). The development of self-representations. In W. Damon (Series Ed.) & N. Eisenberg (Vol. Ed.), *Handbook of child psychology: Vol. 3. Social, emotional, and personality development* (5th ed., pp. 553-617). New York: Wiley.

Hightower, A. D., Cowen, E. L., Spinell, A. P., Lotyczewski, B. S., Guare, J. C., Rohrbeck, C. A., & Brown, L. P. (1987). The Child Rating Scale: Development of a self-rating scale for elementary school children. *School Psychology Review, 16*, 239-255.

Hightower, A. D., Work, W. C., Cowen, E. L., Lotyczewski, B. S., Spinell, A. P., Guare, J. C., & Rohrbeck, C. A. (1986). The Teacher-Child Rating Scale: A brief objective measure of elementary school children's problem behaviors and competencies. *School Psychology Review, 15*, 393-409.

Hodges, E. V. E., Boivin, M., Vitaro, F., & Bukowski, W. M. (1999). The power of friendship: Protection against an escalating cycle of peer victimization. *Developmental Psychology, 35*, 94-101.

Hodges, E. V. E., & Perry, D. G. (1999). Personal and interpersonal antecedents and consequences of victimization by peers. *Journal of Personality and Social Psychology, 7*, 677-685.

Huberty, C. J., & Morris, J. D. (1989). Multivariate analysis versus multiple univariate analyses. *Psychological Bulletin, 105*, 302-308.

Isaacs, J., Card, N. A., & Hodges, E. V. E. (2000, June). *Aggression, peer victimization, social cognitions, and weapon carrying in schools.* Paper presented at the annual meeting of the American Psychological Society, Miami Beach, FL.

Kochenderfer-Ladd, B., & Ladd, G. W. (2001). Variations in peer victimization: Relations to children's maladjustment. In J. Juvonen & S. Graham (Eds.), *Peer harassment in school: The plight of the vulnerable and victimized* (pp. 25-48). New York: Guilford Press.

Kochenderfer, B. J., & Ladd, G. W. (1996). Peer victimization: Cause or consequence of school maladjustment? *Child Development, 67, 1305 1317.*

Kochenderfer-Ladd, B., & Wardrop, J. L. (2001). Chronicity and instability of children's peer victimization experiences as predictors of loneliness and social satisfaction trajectories. *Child Development, 72, 134-151.*

Kovacs, M. (1992). *Children's Depression Inventory (CDI) Manual.* New York: Multi-Health Systems, Inc.

Mynard, H., Joseph, S., & Alexander, J. (2000). Peer victimization and posttraumatic stress in adolescents. *Personality and Individual Differences, 29, 815-821.*

Olweus, D. (1978). *Aggression in the schools: Bullies and whipping boys.* Washington, DC: Hemisphere Press.

Pellegrini, A. D., Bartini, M., & Brooks, F. (1999). School bullies, victims, and aggressive victims: Factors relating to group affiliation and victimization in early adolescence. *Journal of Educational Psychology, 91, 216-224.*

Perry, D. G., Hodges, E. V. E., & Egan, S. K. (2001). Determinants of chronic victimization by peers: A review and a new model of family influence. In J. Juvonen & S. Graham (Eds.), *Peer harassment in school: The plight of the vulnerable and victimized* (pp. 73-104). New York: Guilford Press.

Perry, D. G., Perry, L. C., & Kennedy, E. (1992). Conflict and the development of antisocial behavior. In C. U. Shantz & W. W. Hartup (Eds.), *Conflict in child and adolescent development* (pp. 301-329). New York: Cambridge University Press.

Peterson, L., & Rigby, K. (1999). Countering bullying at an Australian secondary school with students as helpers. *Journal of Adolescence, 22, 481-492.*

Rigby, K. (2000). Effects of peer victimization in schools and perceived social support on adolescent well-being. *Journal of Adolescence, 23, 57-68.*

Schwartz, D., Chang, L., & Farver, J. M. (2001). Correlates of victimization in Chinese children's peer groups. *Developmental Psychology, 37, 520-532.*

Schwartz, D., Dodge, K. A., Pettit, G. S., & Bates, J. E. (1997). The early socialization of aggressive victims of bullying. *Child Development, 68, 665-675.*

Underwood, M. K., Galen B. R., & Paquette, J. A. (2001). Top ten challenges for understanding gender and aggression in children: Why can't we all just get along? *Social Development, 10, 248-266.*

Verkuyten, M., & Thijs, J. (2001). Peer victimization and self-esteem of ethnic minority group children. *Journal of Community and Applied Social Psychology, 11, 227-234.*

The Association of Bullying and Victimization with Middle School Adjustment

Tonja R. Nansel
Denise L. Haynie
Bruce G. Simons-Morton

National Institute of Child Health and Human Development

SUMMARY. Bullying others or being victimized during the transition to middle school may be an important risk factor for school adjustment problems; however, it has been minimally addressed in previous research. This study examined the relationship of bullying and being victimized during the first year of middle school with subsequent school adjustment. Self-report data were obtained from 930 youth at the beginning of 6th grade, the end of 6th grade, and the end of 7th grade. After controlling for baseline scores, youth who were classified as bullies, victims, or bully-victims during sixth grade showed poorer school adjustment than their non-involved peers. In addition, those who were victims or bully-victims during 6th grade reported a more negative perceived school climate than bullies or comparison youth. These differences persisted over time.

Address correspondence to: Tonja R. Nansel, PhD, Division of Epidemiology, Statistics, and Prevention Research, National Institute of Child Health and Human Development, 6100 Executive Boulevard, Room 7B05, MSC 7510, Bethesda, MD 20892-7510 (E-mail: nanselt@mail.nih.gov).

[Haworth co-indexing entry note]: "The Association of Bullying and Victimization with Middle School Adjustment." Nansel, Tonja, Denise L. Haynie, and Bruce G. Simons-Morton. Co-published simultaneously in *Journal of Applied School Psychology* (The Haworth Press, Inc.) Vol. 19, No. 2, 2003, pp. 45-61; and: *Bullying, Peer Harassment, and Victimization in the Schools: The Next Generation of Prevention* (ed: Maurice J. Elias, and Joseph E. Zins) The Haworth Press, Inc., 2003, pp. 45-61. Single or multiple copies of this article are available for a fee from The Haworth Document Delivery Service [1-800-HAWORTH, 9:00 a.m. - 5:00 p.m. (EST). E-mail address: docdelivery@haworthpress.com].

Findings suggest that problematic peer interactions may hinder youth's adaptation to the middle school environment. *[Article copies available for a fee from The Haworth Document Delivery Service: 1-800-HAWORTH. E-mail address: <docdelivery@haworthpress.com> Website: <http://www.HaworthPress. com> © 2003 by The Haworth Press, Inc. All rights reserved.]*

KEYWORDS. Bullying, victimization, school adjustment, school climate, middle school, transition

INTRODUCTION

The transition from elementary to middle school is an important developmental task for early adolescents. It is a time typically characterized by increased academic demand, decreased personal attention in school, increased social stressors, and a shift from adult-focused to peer-focused relationships (Eccles, 1999; Elias, Gara, & Ubriaco, 1985; Lynch & Cicchetti, 1997). An important component of adaptation to middle school is the youth's development of healthy social relationships with peers. Peer relationships may influence school adjustment through both affective and social processes. Youths' peer relationships at school function as either supports or stressors in their adjustment to the demands of a new school environment (Birch & Ladd, 1996; Ladd & Price, 1987; Ladd, Kochenderfer, & Coleman, 1997). Difficulties in peer relationships are associated with negative changes in self-concept and feelings of self-worth (Fenzel, 2000; Haynes, 1990; Wenz-Gross, Siperstein, Untch, & Widaman, 1997), which may impair subsequent school adjustment. Conversely, healthy peer relationships may promote positive school adjustment by creating a sense of relatedness that serves a motivational function for youth in school (Connell & Wellborn, 1991; Hicks & Anderman, 1999; Ryan & Powelson, 1991).

A common maladaptive type of peer interaction among middle-school youth is that of bullying. Bullying is typically defined as aggressive peer-to-peer behavior in which (1) there is an intention to harm or disturb the victim; (2) the aggression occurs repeatedly over time; and (3) there is an imbalance of power, with a more powerful person or group attacking a less powerful one (Olweus, 1993). The aggressive behavior may be verbal (e.g., name-calling, threats), physical (e.g., hitting), or psychological (e.g., rumors, shunning/exclusion). Bullying is a relatively common phenomenon among early adolescents. In a nationally representative study of U.S. youth in grades 6-10, 29.9% reported involvement in moderate or frequent bullying, with 13.0% bullying others, 10.6% being bullied, and 6.3% reporting both bullying others and being bullied. Bullying occurred more frequently among 6th to 8th grade youth than among those in grades 9 and 10 (Nansel, Overpeck, Pilla, Ruan, & Simons-Morton, 2001).

Involvement in bullying during the transition to middle school may represent an important risk factor for subsequent school adjustment. Both bullying others and being victimized represent maladaptive peer relationships, which could predispose the youth to increased difficulty during the middle-school transition. However, the relationship between bullying/victimization and school adjustment has not been adequately addressed in previous research. The purpose of this study was to determine the relationship of bullying and being victimized during the first year of middle school with school adjustment and perceived school climate at the end of the first and second years of middle school. We examined the continuity of bullying behaviors over time, and investigated the extent to which bullies, victims, and bully-victims differed from non-involved youth in their adjustment to middle school.

REVIEW OF RELEVANT LITERATURE

The developmental challenges associated with the transition to middle school may result in personal and academic difficulties for youth. Overall, students typically experience an increase in psychological distress and a decrease in academic motivation and achievement during the transition to middle school (Blyth, Simmons, & Carlton-Ford, 1983; Crockett, Peterson, Graber, Schulenberg, & Ebata, 1989; Gutman & Midgley, 2000; Hirsch & Rapkin, 1987; Simmons & Blyth, 1987; Wigfield, Eccles, MacIver, Reuman, & Midgley, 1991). While these findings occur across racial and socioeconomic status groups, individual students vary in the extent to which they experience such transition difficulties (Chung, Elias, & Schneider, 1996; Crockett et al., 1989; Fenzel & Blyth, 1986; Hirsch & Rapkin, 1987; Simmons & Blyth, 1987). Thus, it is likely that various risk and protective factors may influence the degree of difficulty experienced.

Previous research indicates that one important factor influencing middle school adjustment may be that of the youth's peer relationships. In a predominantly middle-class sample of Canadian youth, McDougall and Hymel (1998) found that transition differences between youth were predicted by both social adjustment and school attitudes/behaviors, with social adjustment playing a potentially critical role. In a study of low-income Black children, adjustment during the first year of middle school was predicted by both aggression and peer rejection (Coie, Lochman, Terry, & Hyman, 1992). Support for various mechanisms linking peer relationships to academic adjustment has been found. One study conducted with youth in a working-class, ethnically diverse Midwestern community, found support for the mediating role of prosocial behavior (Wentzel & Caldwell, 1997). Another conducted with a sample of ethnically diverse urban middle-school youth supported an explanatory model in which peer harassment negatively influences psychological adjustment, which subsequently affects school adjustment (Juvonen, Nishina, & Graham, 2000).

There is much support for the assertion that peer harassment has a negative effect on psychological adjustment. Research conducted across countries and with diverse samples has consistently found that both bullies and victims of bullying demonstrate poorer psychosocial functioning than their non-involved peers. Youth who bully others tend to demonstrate higher levels of conduct problems and externalizing behaviors, whereas youth who are bullied generally show higher levels of internalizing behaviors, including anxiety, depression, loneliness, unhappiness, and low self-esteem, as well as increased physical symptoms (Austin & Joseph, 1996; Boulton & Underwood, 1992; Forero, McLellan, Rissel, & Bauman, 1999; Hawker & Boulton, 2000; Haynie et al., 2001; Hodges & Perry, 1999; Kaltiala-Heino, Rimpela, Rantanen, & Rimpela, 2000; Kumpulainen, Rasanen, & Henttonen, 1999; Nansel et al., 2001; Olweus, 1978; Olweus, 1993; Rigby, 1999; Salmon, James, & Smith, 1998; Williams, Chambers, Logan, & Robinson, 1996). Moreover, youth who both bully others and are victims of bullying demonstrate even poorer psychosocial functioning than youth who only bully or are only victimized (Andreuo, 2000; Austin & Joseph, 1996; Forero et al., 1999; Kaltiala-Heino et al., 2000; Kumpulainen et al., 1998; Haynie et al., 2001; Nansel et al., 2001).

Studies conducted to date, then, suggest that peer relationships influence psychological adjustment, and subsequently, psychological adjustment affects school adjustment. This relationship may be especially acute during the middle-school years, when youth are shifting emphasis from adult-focused to peer-focused relationships. If maladaptive peer relationships do in fact have a negative impact on school adjustment due to their detrimental effect on psychosocial functioning, youth who bully others and youth who are bullied would be at risk for school adjustment problems. This study focuses on bullying that occurs during the sixth grade year–when students are in the middle-school transition period.

METHODS

Participants

Self-report survey data were obtained from two cohorts of students in four middle schools (grades 6-8) in one suburban Maryland school district. The county in which this school district resides is racially diverse, with 69% of residents White, 26% African American, 2% Hispanic and 2% Asian (U.S. Census Bureau, 1990). The 1997 model based estimates for the percent of people of all ages in poverty in the county is 7%, and median income is $54,110, according to the U.S. Census Bureau. Students starting 6th grade in the fall of 1996 and the fall of 1997 were recruited to participate in the study. Special education students with reading disabilities (n = 119) were considered ineligible. Data were obtained in the fall of 6th grade, the spring of 6th grade, and the spring of 7th grade. The four schools had been randomly assigned a non-intervention status as part of a district-wide study evaluating the effects of a school-based program targeting multiple problem behaviors. The school district had no other special interventions occurring in the middle schools at the time of the study, as part of their agreement to be the site for the research. From a total of 1,490 eligible 6th grade students, 1,267 (85%) completed the baseline survey. Nonparticipants included 118 parent refusals, 47 non-returned consent forms, 55 absences on both assessment dates, and 3 incomplete/unusable surveys. Of the 1,267 baseline participants, 939 (74%) were also assessed at the following two time points. Lost to follow-up were 116 students who moved out of the county, 42 parent refusals, 60 non-returned consent forms, 43 absences, 33 who moved to a treatment condition school, 27 who were later classified as special education students, and 7 who failed 6th grade. The final sample comprised 47.1% boys and 52.9% girls. The ethnic composition of the sample was 73.7% White students, 16.7% Black students, and 9.6% students of other racial/ethnic backgrounds.

Procedures

Parents and students were informed that the survey was the measurement component of the intervention evaluation study. Written consent was obtained from all parents of the participating students. Students assent was also obtained. Students completed questionnaires during their home-base classroom, with make-up assessments scheduled the following week for students who were absent on the day of assessment. The survey was administered in each classroom by two trained proctors. Study investigators and project staff served as trainers and team leaders, each supervising several pairs of proctors. Teachers remained in the classroom to supervise student discipline but were otherwise uninvolved in the survey procedures. To ensure confidentiality, students first completed and turned in a cover page that included their name, survey identification number, birth date, and home-base classroom teacher's name. Students' names were not on the questionnaires. The study was reviewed by the National Institute of Child Health and Human Development Institutional Review Board and authorized by representatives of the school district.

Measures

The questionnaire was designed to assess behaviors and attitudes targeted by the intervention program. Measures were either selected or created based on extensive review of the relevant published literature. Prior to implementation in this study, a pilot study (n = 130 sixth-grade students) was conducted to ascertain the readability of items and internal consistency of scales. The survey used in the current study consisted of 116 items assessing student background, psychosocial, school, and parent variables, as well as involvement in problem behaviors, a subset of which included questions about bullying and victimization. For the measures of school adjustment and climate, if a student completed at least 3/5 of the items comprising a scale, the value for any missing items was imputed based on the item mean for students of the same grade and gender. Scale scores were then computed (Kessler, Little, & Groves, 1995). A summary of each measure is provided below.

Bullying. Bullying was assessed by asking "How many times in the last year have you bullied or picked on someone younger, smaller, or weaker (not including your brothers and sisters")? Response categories were 0 = zero, 1 = 1 or 2 times, 2 = 3 to 5 times, and 3 = 6 or more times.

Victimization. Victimization during the last year was assessed by asking how many times the respondent had (a) something taken from them by force or threats, (b) been made to do something they did not want to do, (c) been threatened to be physically hurt, and (d) been actually physically hurt. Response categories were 0 = zero, 1 = 1 or 2 times, 2 = 3 to 5 times, and 3 = 6 or more times.

School Adjustment. This 11-item scale measured the student's adjustment in the activities of school, such as doing well on schoolwork, getting along with classmates, following rules, doing homework, etc. Students rate how well the item describes them on a four-point scale: really true, sort of true, sort of false or really false.

School Climate. This 17-item scale, adapted from Pyper and colleagues (1987), includes items measuring perceived teacher support, rule clarity and enforcement, and student respect for one another. Items are rated from strongly agree to strongly disagree on a 4-point scale.

Analysis

As the focus of this study is on bullying/victimization that occurs during the first year of middle school, students were classified as victims, bullies, bully-victims, or comparisons based on their reports in the spring of 6th grade regarding bullying and victimization during the previous year (i.e., during 6th grade). Victims reported having been victimized three or more times in the past year and having never or rarely (two or fewer times) bullied. Bullies reported bullying others three or more times in the past year and never or rarely having been victimized. Bully-victims reported both having bullied and having been victimized three or more times in the past year. Comparison youth were those who reported no bullying or victimization. Students who reported rarely bullying and/or being victimized were not classified in any of the four groups, as the focus of this study is on repeated bullying and victimization during the first year of middle school. Students missing data on either bullying or victimization measures (n = 9; 0.01%) were excluded from the analysis.

Because bullying behaviors may persist over time (Kumpulainen et al., 1999), students who bullied or were victimized during the first year of middle school may have differed from non-involved youth at baseline (fall of 6th grade). Therefore, potential baseline group differences were assessed by analyses of variance (ANOVAs) conducted on baseline measures of bullying, victimization, school adjustment, and school climate using the four-group classification. To control for these baseline differences, analysis of covariance (ANCOVA) was selected as the analytic technique for subsequent analyses. Analysis of covariance adjusts the means on each dependent variable (school adjustment or climate) to their expected levels if all subjects had scored equally on the covariates (baseline bullying, victimization, and the corresponding school measure) (Tabachnick & Fidel, 1996). A series of ANCOVAs were conducted on spring 6th and 7th grade measures of school adjustment and school climate with baseline bullying, victimization, and the corresponding school measure as covariates.

RESULTS

Variable means, standard deviations, range of responses, coefficient alphas, and correlations are presented in Table 1. As anticipated, school adjustment and perceived school climate showed a mean decrease from fall to spring of 6th grade. In addition, perceived school climate declined further by spring of 7th grade. School adjustment and perceived school climate were positively associated with each other, and negatively associated with bullying and victimization.

A total of 199 students (21.4%) reported being victimized repeatedly (three or more times) during their first year of middle school, 25 (2.7%) reported repeatedly bullying others, and 23 (2.5%) reported both repeatedly bullying others and repeatedly being victimized (Table 2). Almost half of the students (n =

TABLE 1. Ranges, Means, Standard Deviations, and Correlations Among Variables

Variable†	range	alpha	mean	SD	1	2	3	4	5	6	7	8	9	10	11
1. F6 Victimization	0-18	.82	1.27	2.43											
2. S6 Victimization	0-24	.84	1.82	3.16	.37										
3. S7 Victimization	0-24	.84	1.79	3.25	.30	.48									
4. F6 Bullying	0-3	--	.21	.57	.30	.20	.10								
5. S6 Bullying	0-3	--	.28	.64	.15	.16	.18	.21							
6. S7 Bullying	0-3	--	.39	.75	.15	.16	.28	.28	.42						
7. F6 School Adjustment	15-44	.85	35.91	5.81	-.22	-.17	-.17	-.24	-.15	-.10					
8. S6 School Adjustment	11-44	.85	33.68	6.26	-.21	-.29	-.20	-.26	-.22	-.18	.49				
9. S7 School Adjustment	14-44	.78	33.21	5.94	-.19	-.28	-.25	-.28	-.19	-.31	.38	.62			
10. F6 School Climate	23-68	.91	59.50	7.38	-.18	-.12	-.13	-.23	-.14	-.09	.41	.34	.26		
11. S6 School Climate	17-68	.92	54.90	9.22	-.14	-.24	-.19	-.20	-.18	-.16	.29	.52	.38	.49	
12. S7 School Climate	17-68	.92	52.18	9.06	-.13	-.20	-.21	-.17	-.13	-.20	.21	.35	.49	.40	.57

†Notation:
F6   Fall of 6th grade
S6   Spring of 6th grade
S7   Spring of 7th grade

TABLE 2. 6th Grade Bully and Victim Groups' Reports of Bullying and Victimization During 7th Grade

6th Grade Group		7th Grade Group			
	None	Minimal†	Victim	Bully	Bully-Victim
Non-bully/Non-victim	62.5%	25.3%	9.4%	1.9%	1.0%
n = 419‡	(260)	(105)	(39)	(8)	(4)
Victim	23.0%	24.2%	46.0%	2.5%	4.0%
n = 199‡	(46)	(48)	(91)	(5)	(8)
Bully	32.0%	8.0%	8.0%	32.0%	20.0%
n = 25	(8)	(2)	(2)	(8)	(5)
Bully/Victim	0.0%	17.4%	47.8%	8.7%	26.1%
n = 23	(0)	(4)	(11)	(2)	(6)

† Those who bullied and/or were victimized only "once or twice."
‡ Four participants were missing data on bullying/victimization at the spring 7th grade assessment. As such, table percentages are calculated based on an n of 416 on the non-bully/non-victim group and 198 in the victim group.

419, 45.1%) reported no bullying or victimization. In addition, 264 (28.4%) reported bullying and/or being victimized once or twice.

Analysis of the four groups' reported bullying and victimization during 7th grade showed considerable continuity from spring of 6th to spring of 7th grade. (The 6th grade measures were done seven months apart, thus, continuity from fall to spring of 6th grade was not assessed due to overlap in the 12-month time frame of these two measures.) As seen in Table 2, most students who reported no bullying or victimization during 6th grade also reported two or fewer such incidents during 7th grade. About half of the 6th grade victims reported 7th grade victimization and half of the 6th grade bullies reported 7th grade bullying. Among the 6th grade bully-victims, almost all were bullies, victim or both in 7th grade.

A series of ANOVAs for bullying, victimization, school adjustment, and school climate at the fall of 6th grade showed significant baseline differences between the four groups (F = 40.34 for victimization, 18.35 for bullying, 12.38 for school adjustment, and 4.19 for school climate; p < .01 for all variables). That is, students who bullied others and/or were victimized during their first year of middle school were significantly different on these measures when they entered middle school. Therefore, adjusting for baseline scores on these measures is warranted.

The results of the ANCOVAs demonstrated poorer adjustment to middle school at both spring of 6th grade and spring of 7th grade among victims, bullies, and bully-victims after controlling for baseline scores on these measures

(Table 3). Bully and victim group status demonstrated a significant effect on school adjustment and climate at spring of 6th and 7th grade above that explained by baseline scores. Bullies, victims, and bully-victims all demonstrated poorer school adjustment than their non-involved peers even after controlling for their poorer baseline scores on these measures. These differences were present at spring of 6th grade and persisted through spring of 7th grade. Victims and bully-victims also reported a more negative perceived school climate at spring of both 6th and 7th grades than non-involved students.

DISCUSSION

Overview of Findings

Findings from this study indicate that bullying and victimization are common problems among youth. More than one-half of sixth grade youth reported some level of bullying, victimization, or both, and over one-fourth reported repeated bullying and/or victimization. Both bullying and victimization demonstrated continuity over time, with over half of students who were involved in repeated bullying and/or victimization in 6th grade reporting repeated involvement in 7th grade as well. In contrast, among youth not involved in bullying or victimization during 6th grade, almost 12% reported repeated bullying and/or victimization during 7th grade. This suggests that bullying and/or victimization is a continuing problem for youth who are involved in these behaviors during their first year of middle school.

Results of this study suggest that involvement in bullying others or being a victim of bullying may be a risk factor for poorer adjustment to middle school. Youth who were classified as bullies, victims, or bully-victims during 6th grade all reported poorer school adjustment at both spring of 6th grade and spring of 7th grade than their non-involved peers, even after adjusting for their baseline scores on bullying, victimization, and school adjustment. Similarly, those who were victims or bully-victims during 6th grade reported a more negative perceived school climate at spring of both 6th and 7th grade than bullies or comparison youth. These youth were less adapted to middle school upon entry, but showed even poorer later school adjustment than would be expected from their initial scores. This suggests that the failure to develop positive peer relationships may be an issue not only of social and emotional development, but also may hinder adaptation to the middle school environment as well. This effect may be mediated by poorer psychosocial adjustment for both bullies and victims. In addition, for bullies, it may reflect difficulties with the social constraints and limits placed by the school environment. In previous studies, bul-

TABLE 3. Adjusted and Unadjusted Means for Bully and Victim Groups on School Measures at Spring of 6th and 7th Grade

6th Grade Bully and Victim Group	Spring of 6th Grade				Spring of 7th Grade			
	School Adjustment F = 16.63**		School Climate F = 8.69**		School Adjustment F = 15.29**		School Climate F = 5.48**	
	Unadjusted Mean	Adjusted Mean†	Unadjusted Mean†	Adjusted Mean	Unadjusted Mean	Adjusted Mean†	Unadjusted Mean	Adjusted Mean‡
Non-bully/Non-victims	35.57	34.97[a]	56.96	56.37[a]	35.11	34.65[a]	53.74	53.31[a]
Victims	30.70	31.65[b]	51.80	52.70[b]	30.86	31.56[b]	49.73	50.41[b]
Bullies	30.42	30.91[b]	52.30	53.74[ab]	31.00	31.46[b]	50.83	51.85[ab]
Bully/Victims	30.32	32.31[b]	50.00	51.35[b]	29.64	31.21[b]	48.00	48.78[b]

** $p < .01$

† Adjusted for baseline values on victimization, bullying, and school adjustment. Adjusted means reflect the value that would be expected if all subjects had the same scores at baseline.

‡ Adjusted for baseline values on victimization, bully, and school climate. Adjusted means reflect the value that would be expected if all subjects had the same scores at baseline.

[ab] Means with different superscripts are significantly different from each other.

lies have been found to like school less (Rigby & Slee, 1991) and to be less popular with teachers (Slee & Rigby, 1993) than other youth. For victims, the lack of safety in the school environment may also contribute to poorer adjustment to school.

In the past, bullying has often been viewed as a minor problem among youth–as a negative but normative and unavoidable aspect of peer interaction (Arora & Thompson, 1987; Hoover & Oliver, 1996). Findings from the current study add to the body of research indicating that bullying is associated with detrimental outcomes for both bullies and victims. As such, it should be treated as a significant issue for youth, warranting efforts to promote youth and adult norms intolerant of bullying.

Strengths and Limitations

This study is one of the few to address the relationship between bullying and school adjustment over time. The longitudinal nature of the data provides several strengths. Continuity of bullying/victimization over time were assessed. Baseline differences on the variables of interest were controlled for in the analysis, and outcomes were measured during spring of both the first and second years of middle school. Nevertheless, the study's limitations must be recognized as well. Variables associated with bullying and victimization were assessed through self-report, and measures used were brief, as bullying was not the main focus of the survey. Further, the measure of bullying in this study might have tapped primarily direct, aggressive bullying, and not other behaviors, such as teasing or exclusion, which are not as commonly associated with the word "bully." As such, the number of youth in the bully and bully victim groups were small, limiting the power of the study. The youth in this study, while ethnically diverse, were from a primarily suburban area of an eastern city, and may differ from youth in rural or urban areas and those from other parts of the country. Finally, this study did not investigate causes of bullying or potential variables that might account for both bullying/victimization and school adjustment problems (e.g., family socialization, individual character, etc.), nor did it test the potential pathway of the effect of peer harassment on school adjustment through psychological adjustment.

Implications for Research and Practice

While much research has been conducted on aggressive behavior among U.S. youth, little attention has been paid specifically to bullying. However, a large body of international research provides a foundation for future study and intervention in this area (Smith & Brain, 2000). Research conducted in Norway and England has demonstrated that the incidence of bullying in schools can, in fact, be reduced substantially through school-based interventions that create changes within the school and classroom environment (Olweus, 1991; Olweus, 1994; Smith, 1997; Sharp & Smith, 1991). Findings from these studies demonstrate the importance of creating a school environment (1) characterized by warmth, positive interest, and involvement from adults–where students feel they are cared about and expected to do well; and (2) where there are clear, firm limits to peer harassment and bullying that are consistently enforced. Important components of these bullying prevention programs include clear and explicit expectations regarding the treatment of others, the use of classroom meetings addressing peer relationships, the incorporation of activities promoting respect for others into day-to-day curriculum, adequate supervision of youth, adult intervention in bullying situations, individual intervention with bullies and victims as needed, ongoing staff training/development, and the facilitation of parental involvement.

Findings from this study support the need for these types of programs in the U.S. and highlight the importance of early prevention, before these behavior patterns become entrenched, and concomitant adjustment problems occur. Bullying prevention information and materials for educators are becoming increasingly available and may provide a useful start for the promotion of school-based bullying prevention efforts (e.g., Committee for Children, 2001; Froschl, Sprung, & Mullin-Rindler, 1998; Garrity, Jens, Porter, Sager, & Short-Camilli, 2001; Hoover & Oliver, 1996; Olweus, Limber, & Mihalic, 1999). However, as little research has been done on the effectiveness of bullying prevention programs in the U.S., these efforts should include efficacy and effectiveness trials to determine effective and feasible models for U.S. schools. Adaptations of programs based on school size, grade levels served, geographic location, and culture also need to be addressed. In addition, the hypothesized model linking peer relationships to school adjustment through psychological adjustment needs to be more fully tested in future studies. Adjustment to school represents an important task of youth, one that may parallel later adaptation to the work world and other adult responsibilities. Promoting positive peer relationships and preventing abuse and harassment among youth may be an essential element of healthy youth development.

REFERENCES

Anderman, L. H. & Anderman, E. M. (1999). Social predictors of changes in students' achievement goal orientations. *Contemporary Educational Psychology, 24*(1), 21-37.

Andreuo, E. (2000). Bully/victim problems and their association with psychological constructs in 8- to 12-year-old Greek schoolchildren. *Aggressive Behavior, 26*(1), 49-56.

Arora, C. M. & Thompson, D. A. (1987). Defining bullying for a secondary school. *Educational and Child Psychology, 4*(3-4), 110-120.

Austin, S. & Joseph, S. (1996). Assessment of bully/victim problems in 8- to 11-year-olds. *British Journal of Educational Psychology, 66*, 447-456.

Birch, S. H. & Ladd, G. W. (1996). Interpersonal relationships in the school environment and children's early school adjustment: The role of teachers and peers. In J. Juvonen & K. R. Wentzel (Eds.), *Social Motivation: Understanding Children's School Adjustment* (pp. 199-225). Cambridge University Press.

Blyth, D. A., Simmons, R. G., & Carlton-Ford, S. (1983). The adjustments of early adolescents to school transitions. *Journal of Early Adolescence, 3*(1-2), 105-120.

Boulton, M. J. & Underwood, K. (1992). Bully/victim problems among middle school children. *British Journal of Educational Psychology, 62*, 73-87.

Chung, H., Elias, M., & Schneider, K. (1998). Patterns of individual adjustment changes during middle school transition. *Journal of School Psychology, 36*(1), 83-101.

Coie, J. D., Lochman, J. E., Tery, R., & Hyman, C. (1992). Predicting early adolescent disorder from childhood aggression and peer rejection. *Journal of Consulting and Clinical Psychology, 60*(5), 783-792.

Committee for Children (2001). Steps to Respect: A bullying prevention program. Seattle, Washington: Committee for Children. Available at http://www.cfchildren.org/str.html

Connell, J.P., & Wellborn, J.G. (1991). Competence, autonomy, and relatedness: A motivational analysis of self-system processes. In M. R. Gunnar & L.A. Sroufe (Eds.), *Self processes in development: Minnesota Symposium on Child Psychology* (vol. 23, pp. 43-77). Hillsdale, NJ: Erlbaum.

Crockett, L. J., Peterson, A. C., Graber, J. A., Schulenberg, J., & Ebata, A. (1989). School transitions and adjustment during early adolescence. *Journal of Early Adolescence, 9*(3), 181-210.

Eccles, J. S. (1999). The Development of Children Ages 6 to 14. *The Future of Children, 9*(2), 30-44.

Elias, M. J., Gara, M., & Ubriaco, M. (1985). Sources of Stress and Support in Children's Transition to Middle School: An empirical analysis. *Journal of Clinical Child Psychology, 14*(2), 112-118.

Fenzel, L. M. (2000). Prospective study of changes in global self-worth and strain during the transition to middle school. *Journal of Early Adolescence, 20*(1), 93-116.

Fenzel, L. M. & Blyth, D. A. (1986). Individual adjustment to school transitions: An exploration of the role of supportive peer relations. *Journal of Early Adolescence, 6*(4), 315-329.

Forero, R., McLellan, L., Rissel, C., & Bauman, A. (1999). Bullying behaviour and psychosocial health among school students in New South Wales, Australia: Cross-sectional survey. *British Medical Journal, 319*, 344-348.

Froschl, M., Sprung, B., & Mullin-Rindler, N. (1998). Quit it: A teacher's guide on teasing and bullying for use with students in grades K-3. New York: Educational Equity Concepts.

Garrity, C., Jens, K., Porter, W., Sager, N., & Short-Camilli, C. (2001). Bully proofing your school: A comprehensive approach for elementary schools. Longmont, Colorado: Sopris West.

Guttman, L. M., & Midgley, C. (2000). The role of protective factors in supporting the academic achievement of poor African American students during the middle school transition. *Journal of Youth and Adolescence, 29*(2), 223-248.

Hawker, D. S. J. & Boulton, M. J. (2000). Twenty years' research on peer victimization and psychosocial maladjustment: A meta-analytic review of cross-sectional studies. *Journal of Child Psychology and Psychiatry, 41*, 441-455.

Haynes, N. M. (1990). Influence of self-concept on school adjustment among middle-school students. *Journal of Social Psychology, 13*(2), 199-207.

Haynie, D. L., Nansel, T. R., Eitel, P., Crump, A. D., Saylor, K. E., Yu, K., & Simons-Morton, B. G. (2001). Bullies, victims, and bully/victims: Distinct groups of youth at risk. *Journal of Early Adolescence, 21*(1), 29-50.

Hirsch, B. J. & Rapkin, B. D. (1987). The transition to junior high school: A longitudinal study of self-esteem, psychological symptomatology, school life and social support. *Child Development, 58*(5), 1235-1243.

Hodges, E. V. E. & Perry, D. B. (1999). Personal and interpersonal antecedents and consequences of victimization by peers. *Journal of Personality and Social Psychology, 76*(4), 677-685.

Hoover, J. H. & Oliver, R. L. (1996). *The bullying prevention handbook: A guide for principals, teachers, and counselors.* Bloomington, Indiana: National Educational Services.

Juvonen, J., Nishina, A., & Graham, S. (2000). Peer harassment, psychological adjustment, and school functioning in early adolescence. *Journal of Educational Psychology, 92*(2), 349-359.

Kaltiala-Heino, R., Rimpela, M., Rantanen, P., & Rimpela, A. (2000). Bullying at school: An indicator of adolescents at risk for mental disorders. *Journal of Adolescence, 23*(6), 661-674.

Kessler, R. C., Little, R. J. A., & Groves, R. M. (1995). Advances in strategies for minimizing and adjusting for survey nonresponse. *Epidemiologic Reviews, 17*(1), 192-204.

Kumpulainen, K., Rasanen, E., & Henttonen, I. (1999). Children involved in bullying: Psychological disturbance and the persistence of the involvement. *Child Abuse and Neglect, 23*(12), 1253-1262.

Kumpulainen, K., Rasanen, E., Henttonen, I., Almqvist, F., Kresanov, K., Linna, S. L., Moilanen, I., Piha, J., Tamminen, T., & Puura, K. (1998). Bullying and psychiatric symptoms among elementary school-age children. *Child Abuse and Neglect, 22*(7), 705-717.

Ladd, G. W., Kochenderfer, B. J., & Coleman, C. C. (1997). Classroom peer acceptance, friendship, and victimization: Distinct relational systems that contribute uniquely to a children's school adjustment? *Child Development, 68*(6), 1181-1197.

Ladd, G. W., & Price, J. M. (1987). Predicting children's social and school adjustment following the transition from preschool to kindergarten. *Child Development, 58*(5), 1168-1189.

Lynch, M. & Cicchetti, D. (1997). Children's relationships with adults and peers: An examination of elementary and junior high school students. *Journal of School Psychology, 35*(1), 81-99.

McDougall, P. & Hymel, S. (1998). Moving into middle school: Individual differences in the transition experience. *Canadian Journal of Behavioural Science, 30*(2), 108-120.

Nansel, T. R., Overpeck, M., Pilla, R. S., Ruan, W. J., & Simons-Morton, B. G. (2001). Bullying behaviors among US youth: Prevalence and association with psychosocial adjustment. *Journal of the American Medical Association, 285*(16), 2094-2100.

Olweus, D. (1978). *Aggression in the schools, bullies and whipping boys.* Washington, DC: Hemisphere Publishing Corporation.

Olweus, D. (1993). *Bullying at school: What we know and what we can do.* Oxford: Blackwell.

Olweus, D. (1994). Bullying at school: Long-term outcomes for the victims and an effective school-based intervention program. In L. R. Huesmann (Ed.), *Aggressive behavior: Current perspectives* (pp. 97-130). New York: Plenum Press.

Olweus, D., Limber, S., & Mihalic, S. F. (1999). Blueprints for violence prevention, book nine: Bullying prevention program. Boulder, CO: Center for the Study and Prevention of Violence.

Pellegrini, A. D. (1998). Bullies and victims in school: A review and call for research. *Journal of Applied Developmental Psychology, 19*(2), 165-176.

Pyper, J. R., Freiberg, H. J., Ginsburg, M., & Spuck, D. W. (1987). *Instruments to measure teacher, parent, and student perceptions of school climate.* Bloomington, ID: Phi Delta Kappa.

Rigby, K. (1999). Peer victimisation at school and the health of secondary school students. *British Journal of Educational Psychology, 69,* 95-104.

Rigby, K. & Slee, P. T. (1991). Dimensions of interpersonal relations among Australian children and implications for psychological well-being. *The Journal of Social Psychology, 133*(1), 33-42.

Ryan, R. M. & Powelson, C. L. (1991). Autonomy and relatedness as fundamental to motivation and education. *Journal of Experimental Education, 60*(1), 49-66.

Salmon, G., James, A., & Smith, D. M. (1998). Bullying in schools: Self-reported anxiety, depression, and self-esteem in secondary school children. *British Medical Journal, 317,* 924-925.

Sharp, S. & Smith, P. K. (1991). Bullying in UK schools: The DES Sheffield Bullying Project. *Early Child Development & Care, 77,* 47-55.

Simmons, R. G. & Blyth, D. A. (1987). *Moving into adolescence: The impact of pubertal change and school context.* New York: Aldine.

Slee, P. T. & Rigby, K. (1993a). Australian school children's self-appraisal of interpersonal relations: The bullying experience. *Child Psychiatry and Human Development, 23*(4), 273-282.

Smith, P. K. (1997). Bullying in schools: The UK experience and the Sheffield Anti-Bullying Project. *The Irish Journal of Psychology, 18,* 191-201.

Smith, P. K. & Brain, P. (2000). Bullying in schools: Lessons from two decades of research. *Aggressive Behavior, 26*(1), 1-9.

Tabachnick, B. G. & Fidel, L. S. (1996). *Using multivariate statistics.* New York: Harper Collins.

U.S. Census Bureau (1990). Charles County, Maryland: 1990 Census population, demographic, and housing information. Available at http://quickfacts.census.gov/ cgi-bin/cnty_QuickLinks?24017. Availability verified August 8, 2002.

Wentzel, K. R. & Caldwell, K. (1997). Friendships, peer acceptance, and group membership: Relations to academic achievement in middle school. *Child Development, 68*(6), 1198-1209.

Wenz-Gross, M , Siperstein, G. N., Untch, A. S., & Wldaman, K. F. (1997). Stress, social support, and adjustment of adolescents in middle school. *Journal of Early Adolescence, 17*(2), 129-151.

Wigfield, A., Eccles, J. S., Maclver, D., Reuman, D., & Midgley, C. (1991). Transitions during early adolescence: Changes in children's domain specific self-perceptions and general self-esteem across the transition to junior high school. *Developmental Psychology, 27,* 552-565.

Williams, K., Chambers, M., Logan, S., & Robinson, D. (1996). Association of common health symptoms with bullying in primary school children. *British Medical Journal, 313,* 17-19.

Perceptions and Attitudes Toward Bullying in Middle School Youth: A Developmental Examination Across the Bully/Victim Continuum

Susan M. Swearer
Paulette Tam Cary

University of Nebraska-Lincoln

SUMMARY. We examined middle school students' attitudes and perceptions of bullying during their middle school years. Participants were categorized along the bully/victim continuum as bullies, victims, bully-victims, and no-status students based on their self-nomination from a survey that queries students about their experiences with bullying (either as a bully, victim, or both), their observations of bullying, and their attitudes toward bullying. The majority of participants were classified as bullies, victims, and bully-victims as 70% of the participants reported involvement with bullying and/or victimization during their middle school years. Participants' perceptions about bullying and attitudes toward bullying were examined at three points in time. Participants' attitudes toward bullying became more supportive of bullying as students

Address correspondence to: Susan Swearer, Department of Educational Psychology, The University of Nebraska-Lincoln, 40 Teachers College Hall, Lincoln, NE 68588-0345 (E-mail: sswearer@unlserve.unl.edu).

[Haworth co-indexing entry note]: "Perceptions and Attitudes Toward Bullying in Middle School Youth: A Developmental Examination Across the Bully/Victim Continuum." Swearer, Susan M., and Paulette Tam Cary. Co-published simultaneously in *Journal of Applied School Psychology* (The Haworth Press, Inc.) Vol. 19, No. 2, 2003, pp. 63-79; and: *Bullying, Peer Harassment, and Victimization in the Schools: The Next Generation of Prevention* (ed: Maurice J. Elias, and Joseph E. Zins) The Haworth Press, Inc., 2003, pp. 63-79. Single or multiple copies of this article are available for a fee from The Haworth Document Delivery Service [1-800-HAWORTH, 9:00 a.m. - 5:00 p.m. (EST). E-mail address: docdelivery@haworthpress.com].

progressed through middle school. Additionally, external attributes for bullying were cited across all four status groups as reasons for involvement in bullying. Implications for prevention and intervention programs that address bullying are discussed. *[Article copies available for a fee from The Haworth Document Delivery Service: 1-800-HAWORTH. E-mail address: <docdelivery@ haworthpress.com> Website: <http://www.HaworthPress.com> © 2003 by The Haworth Press, Inc. All rights reserved.]*

KEYWORDS. Bullying, victimization, attitudes, peer aggression, adolescence

Bullying, including both verbal and physical behaviors, may be the most prevalent type of school violence (Batsche, 1997). Reported incidence rates, with populations from the United States, range from a conservative 10% for "extreme victims" of bullying (Perry, Kusel, & Perry, 1988) to a high of 75% of school-aged children who reported being bullied at least one time during their school years (Hoover, Oliver, & Hazler, 1992). More recent studies within the United States have found 8.4% (Nansel, Overpeck, Pilla, Ruan, Simons-Morton, & Scheidt, 2001) to 20% (Limber & Small, 2000) of children reporting being victimized several times per week while 24.2% (Nansel et al.) to 44.6% (Haynie et al., 2001) report being bullied at least once during the past year. Recent rates of bullying other students are less variable; approximately 9% (Nansel et al.) to 13% (Limber & Small) of students report bullying other students several times per week while 24% (Nansel et al.) to 25% (Haynie et al.) report bullying other students at least once in the past year.

Within the last decade, the phenomenon of bullying has been recognized as a serious problem for the quality of school life among children (Berthold & Hoover, 2000). Data from the Centers for Disease Control and Prevention Youth Risk Behavior Surveillance survey indicated that 7.4% of American youth reported having been threatened or injured with a weapon on school grounds one or more times within the past year (Kann et al., 1998). In addition, 4% reported missing school within the last 30 days because they feared being intimidated or bullied. Hoover et al. (1992) found that a significant number of victims reported experiencing social and academic trauma resulting from bullying. Batsche and Knoff (1994) reported that victims commonly respond to bullying through escape/avoidance behaviors, such as not going to school, refusing to go to certain places, running away from home, and in some extreme cases, attempting suicide.

Studies have documented that children involved in the bully/victim continuum experience impaired psychosocial functioning (Bosworth, Espelage, &

Simon, 1999; Juvonen, Nishina, & Graham, 2000). Research has found that victims experience impaired physical and mental health (Rigby, 1999), internalizing problems (Swearer, Song, Cary, Eagle, & Mickelson, 2001), and psychosomatic symptoms (Kumpulainen et al., 1998). On the other end of the continuum, bullies report feelings of depression (Kaltiala-Heino et al.; Swearer et al.), and suicidal ideation and behavior (Bailey, 1994; Kaltiala-Heino et al.). Students who both bully others and are bullied (bully-victims) experience psychological distress (Duncan, 1999); anxiety (Craig, 1998); loneliness (Forero, McLellan, Rissel, & Bauman, 1999); and depression (Craig; Kaltiala-Heino, Rimpela, Marttunen, Rimpela, & Rantanen, 1999; Swearer et al.). In fact, these youth may be the most impaired subgroup along the bully/victim continuum (Swearer et al.).

Bullying and victimization appear to pose negative consequences not only at the time they occur within a youth's life, but also, potentially, for their future. Potential long-term negative effects for bullies include an increased risk for becoming involved in delinquent and criminal activity (Loeber & Dishion, 1983; Olweus, 1993). Victims of bullying are more at risk for symptoms of depression and low self-esteem as young adults than compared to their nonvictimized peers (Olweus).

Researchers have suggested that bullying behavior tends to peak in middle school and generally decreases with age (Hoover et al., 1992; Pellegrini & Bartini, 2000). Pellegrini and Bartini note that the increase in bullying behavior occurs when students make the transition into middle school. Thus, bullying behaviors appear to reflect the needs of students to establish social status as they transition into a new peer group. In addition to transitioning into new peer groups, early adolescence is also a time when cross-sex contacts and interactions become an important goal. Breaking the well-established norms of same-sex interactions from early childhood can prove risky; therefore, young adolescents may try to minimize the risks by using playful and/or ambiguous overtures, such as pushing, poking, and teasing, which can be interpreted as bullying (Pellegrini, 2001). Additionally, this study found that sexual harassment in seventh grade was predicted by bullying in sixth grade (Pellegrini).

With the plethora of potential negative consequences resulting from bullying and victimization (e.g., internalizing psychopathology, delinquent pathways, sexual harassment), examining the cognitions and attitudes of students toward bullying may assist researchers and educators in the effort toward developing effective prevention and intervention programs that reduce bullying behaviors. This information may help illustrate the reasons why some students bully and why others do not, as well as identify any beliefs that may contribute to or perpetuate the bullying phenomenon among school-aged youth.

One of the first studies exploring students' perceptions towards bullying was conducted by Olweus (1978). Olweus found that rather than being bullied due to prototypical "nerd" or social-outcast characteristics (e.g., wore glasses, different clothing, spoke differently, overweight, etc.), students were bullied because they appeared physically and/or emotionally weak. Rigby and Slee (1991) found that the majority of Australian children were opposed to bullying and tended to support the victims; however, the children's attitudes toward victims became less supportive as they became older. Specifically, they tended to dislike victims of bullying and admire the bullies. More recently, Rigby (1997) found that as Australian students matured, up to the age of 16, their attitudes became more supportive of bullying, and they reported more participation in bullying. Additionally, males tended to possess more pro-bullying attitudes than females. Similarly, a large-scale survey study from Italy and England found that in both countries the majority of children were opposed to bullying and supportive toward victims with females tending to be more distressed by bullying than males (Menesini et al., 1996). Bullies were found to be more inclined to understand other bullies, feel less sympathetic toward victims' suffering, less likely to intervene when witnessing a bullying episode, and more likely to join in bullying other children they did not like.

Within the United States, Oliver, Hoover, and Hazler (1994) surveyed middle and high school students in Midwestern schools. They found that 64% of students tended to agree that victims brought on teasing themselves, 51% of students felt that teasing was done in fun, and 39% of students felt that bullying "helped" the victim by making him or her tougher. Additionally, when compared to males, 34% of females believed that bullies had higher social status than victims (compared to 24% of males). In an earlier study examining victim characteristics, physical weakness was significantly more likely to motivate bullying if the victim was male while the victims' peer group was more likely to motivate bullying if the victim was female (Hazler, Hoover, & Oliver, 1991). Males have been found to engage in bullying behavior more frequently than girls, while girls have been found to hold more negative attitudes towards bullying than boys (Hazler et al., 1991; Pellegrini & Bartini, 2000).

Pellegrini, Bartini, and Brooks (1999) found that bullies possessed more positive attitudes towards bullying than other groups (i.e., victims and controls). More recently, Pellegrini and Bartini (2000) found that cognitions about bullying did not predict bullying status; therefore, these researchers suggested that positive attitudes toward bullying, especially among bullies, may serve as a strategy to reduce the cognitive dissonance associated with feelings that are inconsistent with the dominant peer and/or cultural norms. However, while this study examined attitudes toward bullying among bullies, victims, and aggressive victims, students who did not experience bullying were not included.

Previous research has documented some patterns of beliefs and attitudes about bullying that students may hold. However, research examining the attitudes and perceptions toward bullying along the bully/victim continuum including not only bullies and victims, but also bully-victims and students not involved in bullying has not been conducted. The purpose of this study was to examine the attitudes and perceptions of middle school students about bullying and to examine attitudes toward bullying across bullies, victims, bully-victims, and students who are neither bullies nor victims (i.e., no status). This study investigated the attitudes and perceptions of students toward bullying throughout their middle-school years, the time in which bullying behavior has been found to peak.

Data were collected over the first three years of a five-year longitudinal study examining ecological factors in bullying in middle-school youth. Ecological factors examined in the larger study include internal psychological factors (depression, anxiety, hopelessness, aggression, locus of control), school climate, teacher and peer nominations of bullies and victims, and prosocial behaviors. Data are presented on the attitudes toward the value of bullying, perceptions of bullying behaviors, and the reasons youth cite for their bullying behaviors across the bully-victim continuum. It was predicted that attitudes supportive of bullying would be associated with external attributions for bullying and that these attitudes would differ across the bully/victim continuum. Additionally, it was predicted that attitudes toward bullying would become more positive as students progressed through middle school.

METHOD

All students at a Midwestern middle school (grades 6 through 8) were eligible to participate in a longitudinal study of bullying and victimization. A letter describing the study, that was signed by the principal investigator and the principal of the school, was sent to all parents of sixth-grade students along with the parental consent form. Active parental consent and youth assent were obtained for each participant in the study. Students in cohort 1, with parental consent to participate in the study, were administered a series of instruments during April 1999 (6th grade), April 2000 (7th grade), and April 2001 (8th grade). Students in cohort 2, with parental consent to participate in the study, were administered a series of instruments during April 2000 (6th grade) and April 2001 (7th grade). The Bully Survey was administered in the spring of every year so that participants had time to get to know their classmates. Results from responses on a survey of bullying and victimization were examined to elucidate changes in perceptions and attitudes toward bullying that students reported throughout middle school.

Participants

Data are presented from sixth-, seventh-, and eighth-grade students in one middle school. In April 1999, 83 sixth-grade students (36 male and 47 female) participated in the study. This reflects at 41% participation rate. Out of the original 83 participants, 66 seventh-grade students (33 male and 33 female) continued in the study. In eighth grade, 57 students (28 male and 29 female) continued in the study. In all cases, when students did not continue in the study, it was due to moving to another school. In April 2000, 50 sixth-grade students (29 male and 21 female) participated in the study. This reflects a 29% participation rate. One hypothesis for this lower participation rate is that the increased media attention to school violence and bullying that occurred after the school shooting in Colorado made parents wary of participating in research on bullying. In fact, several parents expressed concern over allowing their child to participate in a study on bullying. Of these 50 participants, 40 seventh-grade students (21 male and 19 female) continued in the study. Again, the students who did not continue in the study moved to other schools. All participants were assigned a code number to maintain confidentiality, and these code numbers were used to track the data across the three points in time. Thus, 133 sixth-grade, 106 seventh-grade, and 57 eighth-grade students participated in this study.

Demographic characteristics for the participants across grades included, ages ranging from 11-13 years old ($M = 11.67$; $SD = .55$; $n = 133$) for the sixth graders; 12-14 years old ($M = 12.60$; $SD = .58$; $n = 106$) for the seventh graders; and 13-15 years old ($M = 13.54$; $SD = .54$; $n = 57$) for the eighth-grade students. The racial distribution across cohorts was: 64% Caucasian, 14% African-American, 9% Asian/Asian-American, 6% Latino(a), 5% Biracial, 1% Eastern European, and 1% Middle Eastern. These demographic characteristics are consistent with the overall school population.

Participants were grouped according to status (i.e., bully, bully-victim, victim, or no status) based on ratings from their responses on the Bully Survey (see Table 1). In sixth grade the bully/victim distribution was 5% bullies ($n = 7$); 39% victims ($n = 52$); 30% bully-victims ($n = 40$); and 26% no status (i.e., does not experience victimization and/or bullying others) ($n = 34$). In seventh grade the bully/victim distribution was 6% bullies ($n = 6$); 43% victims ($n = 46$); 20% bully-victims ($n = 21$); and 31% no status ($n = 33$). In eighth grade the bully/victim distribution was 7% bullies ($n = 4$); 40% victims ($n = 23$); 21% bully-victims ($n = 12$); and 32% no status ($n = 18$).

TABLE 1. Bully/Victim Status Across Year

	Time 1 (6th)		Time 2 (7th)		Time 3 (8th)	
	%	n	%	n	%	n
Status						
Bully	5%	7	6%	6	7%	4
Victim	39%	52	43%	46	40%	23
Bully-Victim	30%	40	20%	21	21%	12
No Status	26%	34	31%	33	32%	18
Total		133		100		57

Instrumentation

The Bully Survey (Swearer, 2001).[1] The Bully Survey is a three-part, 31-question survey that queries students regarding their experiences with bullying, perceptions of bullying, and attitudes toward bullying during the school year in which the survey is administered. The Bully Survey was developed and pilot tested in 1998 with a 6th grade cohort ($n = 169$), including both regular and special education students. The survey was based on other well-known surveys of bullying; however, items were also included that were of interest to the local school district. Since 1998, the Bully Survey has been used in three middle schools in the Midwest and in a school district in Virginia. It has also been used internationally in Germany, Guatemala, and Peru.

Bullying is defined in each section of the survey as: "Bullying is anything from teasing, saying mean things, or leaving someone out of a group, to physical attacks (hitting, pushing, kicking) where one person or a group of people picks on another person over a long time. Bullying refers to things that happen in school, on the school grounds, or going to and from school." In Part A of the survey, students answered questions about when they were victims of bullying during the past year. Additionally, there are two questions in Part A that ask students if they have experienced bullying at home. If the participants reported they had not been victims of bullying, they were instructed to skip Part A and begin Part B. Part B of the survey addressed questions about the participants' observations of bullying behavior among their peers during the past year. If they reported that they had not observed bullying behavior, the participants were instructed to skip Part B. Part C of the survey requested information from the participants about when they bullied other students. If the participants indicated that they had not bullied other students within the last year, they skipped Part C and completed the final section of the survey. The final section of the survey contained a scale that measures attitudes toward bullying. In the present study, the internal consistency reliability using coefficient alpha was .69 for the total attitude score for Time 1, .55 for Time 2, and .74 for Time 3.

RESULTS

Results will be described in terms of examining perceptions and attitudes toward bullying among bullies, victims, bully-victims, and no status students across their middle school years. SPSS version 10.1 was used to analyze the data.

Given that previous research has found differences between males and females regarding bullying behaviors, analyses were run to determine whether gender differences existed across status groups. Interestingly, there were no differences across status with respect to gender in 6th grade ($\chi^2 = 4.46$, $p = .21$), 7th grade ($\chi^2 = 1.33, p = .72$), and 8th grade ($\chi^2 = 1.33, p = .85$). This suggests that within this sample, there were no differences between boys and girls across status groups (bullies, victims, bully-victim, and no-status participants) during middle school.

An integrity check of the status groups was conducted in order to validate participants' status as reported on the Bully Survey. We examined office referral data across the four status groups across their middle-school years (see Table 2). Students in this school receive office referrals for insubordination, violation of school rules, physical aggression, and verbal aggression. As expected, on average across the middle-school years, bullies had the highest number of office referrals, followed by bully-victims, no-status students, and victims. These data also serve as an indicator of the validity of the Bully Survey, reflecting the fact that students who bully others are more likely to be sent to the office as a disciplinary measure.

Students' experiences with bullying and victimization across their middle school years were examined. Specifically, perceptions regarding the top locations where bullying was reported, who was involved in the bullying, if students were bullied at home, how students felt the school responded to the bullying, and participants' attitudes toward bullying are presented.

Main Locations Where Bullying Occurred

The top three locations across status groups where students felt that bullying occurred are reported (see Table 3). The majority of students across the status groups reported that bullying occurred most frequently in classrooms, hallways, after school, and gym or recess. Across all three years, bully-victims endorsed more locations than the other groups.

TABLE 2. Office Referrals Across Status and Year

Status	Time 1 (6th)		Time 2 (7th)		Time 3 (8th)	
	M	SD	M	SD	M	SD
Bully	1.43	2.15	4.83	4.50	7.75	4.57
Victim	.69	1.45	3.15	5.89	2.87	4.35
Bully-Victim	2.67	5.27	4.50	7.16	6.17	7.77
No Status	3.00	5.77	3.37	8.78	1.24	1.64

Who Was Involved in Bullying Incidents?

Tables 4 and 5 summarize who students report are involved in bullying. It appears that bullying includes a power differential (older students bullying younger students) and that bullying occurs equally among males and females. Bullying is a ubiquitous phenomenon occurring across grade, gender, status, and year.

Perceptions of Bullying

Students' perceptions of why they were bullied or why they bullied others were examined across sixth, seventh, and eighth grades. Interestingly, there was some consistency across status groups concerning students' perceptions of why the bullying behaviors occurred. External attributes such as being different, being weak, and wearing certain clothes were cited across all four status groups as reasons for bullying. Bullies endorsed perceived physical attributes such as the way someone talks, the clothes they wear, or being weak as reasons for bullying. Victims endorsed getting good grades, being weak, overweight, different, and wearing certain clothes as reasons for being bullied. Bully-victims endorsed the same reasons as victims for being bullied and the same reasons for being bullied as a rationale to bully others. No-status students endorsed being weak, overweight, different, and wearing certain clothes as reasons for students being bullied.

Congruence Between Bullying at School and Being Bullied at Home

We were also interested in knowing whether or not students who experienced bullying at school were also bullied at home. Approximately 70% of the victims across all three points in time reported that they were not bullied at home, while bully-victims reported being bullied at home by their siblings (53%; 6th grade), (28%; 7th grade), and (50%; 8th grade).

TABLE 3. Main Locations Participants Reported Bullying to Occur

Location	Time 1 (6th)				Time 2 (7th)				Time 3 (8th)			
	Bully	Victim	Bully-Victim*	No Status	Bully	Victim	Bully-Victim*	No Status	Bully	Victim	Bully-Victim*	No Status
Classroom	43% (#1)	15% (#3)	28% (#1) 15% (#2)	32% (#1)	17% (#2)	11%	35% (#1) 10% (#3)	0%	25% (#3)	39% (#2)	25% 17%	42% (#2)
Hallway	29% (#2)	19% (#1)	20% (#2) 15% (#2)	16% (#2)	0%	41% (#1)	20% (#2) 14% (#2)	29% (#1)	50% (#2)	61% (#1)	67% (#1) 42% (#1)	58% (#1)
After School	14% (#3)	17% (#2)	8% 18% (#1)	11%	0%	15% (#2)	10% 5%	18% (#2)	75% (#1)	30%	42% (#2) 25%	33% (#3)
Gym	14% (#3)	10%	3% 15% (#2)	11%	33% (#1)	15% (#2)	15% (#3) 4% (#2)	6%	50% (#2)	35% (#3)	33% (#3) 33% (#2)	25%
Recess	0%	14%	13% (#3) 5%	16% (#3)	17% (#2)	15% (#2)	20% (#2) 24% (#1)	12% (#3)	25% (#3)	26%	33% (#3) 33% (#2)	25%
Cafeteria	0%	12%	8% 8% (#3)	5%	0%	13% (#3)	20% (#2) 4% (#2)	12% (#3)	50% (#2)	30%	17% 8%	58% (#1)

*Note: Locations where bully-victims reported bullying others are listed first, followed by where bully-victims reported being victimized.

TABLE 4. Victims as Reported by Bullies and Bully-Victims

Victims	Time 1 (6th)		Time 2 (7th)		Time 3 (8th)	
	Bullies	Bully-Victims	Bullies	Bully-Victims	Bullies	Bully-Victims
Younger Boys	71%	45%	67%	43%	0%	33%
Younger Girls	71%	43%	67%	38%	0%	33%
Same Grade Boys	57%	63%	83%	62%	50%	75%
Same Grade Girls	57%	55%	33%	38%	50%	58%
Older Boys	43%	45%	67%	38%	25%	17%
Older Girls	57%	40%	33%	33%	0%	8%

TABLE 5. Bullies as Reported by Victims, Bully-Victims, and No-Status Students

Bullies	Time 1 (6th)			Time 2 (7th)			Time 3 (8th)		
	Victims	Bully-Victims	No Status	Victims	Bully-Victims	No Status	Victims	Bully-Victims	No Status
Younger Boys	19%	35%	42%	24%	29%	47%	0%	8%	17%
Younger Girls	28%	30%	42%	20%	14%	35%	0%	17%	17%
Same-Grade Boys	48%	50%	74%	59%	62%	71%	67%	33%	92%
Same-Grade Girls	52%	43%	58%	37%	29%	59%	30%	42%	42%
Older Boys	60%	60%	53%	48%	62%	71%	22%	8%	25%
Older Girls	44%	33%	47%	30%	33%	47%	9%	0%	17%

Perceptions of the Schools' Response to Bullying

Across all three points in time, bullies, victims, and no-status students felt that when school staff knew the bullying occurred, they responded in a satisfactory fashion. However, bully-victims felt that the school did not address bullying issues well (when they were either victims or bullies). The majority of the sample across their middle school years felt that schools should worry about bullying (80%). However, 80% of the sample reported that the school staff did not know that the bullying occurred.

Attitudes Toward Bullying Across Middle School

Over time, the participants' attitudes toward bullying were fairly consistent with a trend towards having more favorable attitudes toward bullying by the eighth grade. There were significant differences between groups on attitudes toward bullying in 7th and 8th grades. In 7th grade, victims had less favorable attitudes toward bullying than the bullies or the no-status students ($F = 3.35; p = .02$). In 8th grade, victims had less favorable attitudes toward bullying than the bully-victims ($F = 2.65; p = .05$).

DISCUSSION

Several interesting patterns emerged from the current study. Specifically, there were no differences in terms of gender across bullies, victims, bully-victims, and no-status groups. When one considers our use of the definition of bullying that includes both verbal and physical behaviors, this finding is consistent with previous research that has found that girls and boys are equally involved in bullying when bullying includes both overt and covert behaviors (Ahmad & Smith, 1994; Boulton & Smith, 1994; Hoover et al., 1992) and that students include both verbal and physical aggression in their definition of bullying (Espelage & Asidao, 2001).

When asked about the location of bullying incidents, most participants reported that they were bullied in more than one location in and around the school building. Bullying was reported to occur most frequently in hallways, academic classrooms, gym and/or recess, and after school. This is consistent with previous research that has found bullying occurs in those same locations (Limber & Small, 2000). This finding has implications for program development, as schools can implement interventions such as increasing the number of hall monitors, monitoring the school grounds, and adopting teacher training programs that help teachers identify bullying behaviors.

In examining the participants' reports of who is involved in bullying incidents, it appears that both boys and girls are equally involved in bullying incidents over the three years. Previous research suggests that the relationship between predictor variables such as school and family functioning are similar for boys and girls (Haynie et al., 2001). Thus, while the forms of bullying may look different in boys and girls, the phenomenon of bullying may occur consistently across gender and grade.

Open-ended responses on the bully survey were examined to add a descriptive element to the perceptions and attitudes that the participants reported. Several of the bullies commented that they bullied other students in response to internal feelings they were experiencing (e.g., "bullying releases my stress" and "when I have a bad day I feel like I need to pick on someone"). Bullies also acknowledged that bullying "proves I'm stronger" and they bully to "fit in." Bullies also stated that they bully others "because they hate me" and "they were making fun of me and talking behind my back." Internal factors have been hypothesized to be related to erroneous attributional style in youth who are aggressive toward others (Dodge & Frame, 1982). In situations where the social interaction is actually neutral, aggressive youth have been found to interpret those interactions as hostile (Dodge, 1993). Some of these comments underscore the research that has examined reasons behind bullying and aggressive behavior in youth and suggest that interventions that target cognitive distortions may be best directed toward bullies and bully-victims.

Victims' open-ended comments support research findings that have concluded that victims are persecuted for external attributions (Bernstein & Watson, 1997; Hazler et al., 1991; Ma, 2001). Victims stated that they are bullied because "I am fat," "I'm smarter than a lot of people," "how I dress," "how I look," and "because of my teeth." As expected, in this study, victims and no-status students held the least favorable attitudes toward bullying. Thus, interventions that include social perspective-taking and that include both victims and bystanders may be important prevention and intervention components.

Bully-victims in this study report that they are also bullied at home and that their siblings are the primary perpetrators of the bullying. Previous research has found that youth with more siblings are more likely to bully others in the school setting (Eslea & Smith, 2000; Ma, 2001). While we did not examine family constellation, it would be interesting to determine if bully-victims come from larger families. The bully-victims' open-ended responses were associated with feelings of getting even. For example, "They bullied me, so I bullied them." Given the connection to being bullied at home for bully-victims, this could be associated with sibling relationships where issues of fairness may be prevalent.

Participants in this study began middle school in the 6th grade. According to Pellegrini and Bartini (2000), bullying may serve a function of establishing dominance and may assist students in the transition to middle school. Because the grade in which students transition to middle school differs across school districts, school administrators and staff may wish to focus on intervention efforts for students in their first year of middle school. This may be the most difficult year in terms of bullying for middle-school youth.

This study represents part of a larger longitudinal study examining bullying and victimization in middle-school youth and is not without limitations. First, we examined self-report data for attitudes and perceptions of bullying for which we do not have external data to validate the participants' responses. For example, we validated status by examining office referral data from school records; however, we could not validate attitudes toward bullying by using another source of data. Second, the cell sizes in this data set continue to be small which precludes submitting these data to more rigorous statistical analyses. Another problem related to cell size is the inability to examine differences across status by gender. When these analyses were conducted, the cell sizes were too small to make meaningful conclusions. Finally, these data were collected from one Midwestern middle-school and thus cannot be generalized to other populations.

Implications for Practice and Policy

Results suggest that an important element of bullying prevention and intervention programs should include components that address perceptions and attitudes toward bullying. Additionally, teacher and staff training programs should include training on the complexity behind bullying behaviors. The participants in this study stated that school staff typically did not know that the bullying had occurred. This is consistent with research that has found that students do not feel the school staff is interested in reducing bullying (Harris, Petrie, & Willoughby, 2002). If students feel that the school staff does not care about bullying or that the staff is unaware that bullying occurs, then they may not feel hopeful that these behaviors can change.

Many state legislatures are mandating that schools adopt anti-bullying policies. While policies are helpful to standardize procedures for responding to problems, schools must be given the tools and the financial support to implement these policies. Schools must also be partners with researchers to conduct research on bullying in their unique school ecology. Each school ecology is unique, and effective research that can be translated into effective practice should guide the development and implementation of prevention and intervention programs.

Bullying should be viewed as an interaction between the individual and his or her peers, school, family, culture, and community (Swearer & Doll, 2001). This definition of bullying presumes an ecological understanding of the phenomenon. Thus, bullying is not simply a behavior, and the titles of "bully" "victim" and "bully-victim" do not represent an innate characteristic of a person. Results from this study reinforce this framework by examining bullying behaviors utilizing a comprehensive assessment of perceptions and attitudes toward bullying. As researchers, educators, and youth begin to understand the complexities behind bullying, inclusion of ecological contexts will help guide effective intervention and prevention programs.

NOTE

1. The Bully Survey (Swearer, 2001) can be obtained from the first author.

REFERENCES

Ahmad, Y. & Smith, P. K. (1994). Bullying in schools and the issue of sex differences. In J. Archer (Ed.), *Male violence* (pp. 70-83). London: Routledge.

Bailey, S. (1994). Health in young persons' establishments: Treating the damaged and preventing harm. *Criminal Behavior and Mental Health, 3*, 349-367.

Batsche, G. M. (1997). Bullying. In G. G. Bear, K. M. Minke, & A. Thomas (Eds.), *Children's Needs II: Development, Problems, and Alternatives* (pp. 171-179). Bethesda, MD: National Association of School Psychologists.

Batsche, G. M. & Knoff, H. M. (1994). Bullies and their victims: Understanding a pervasive problem in the schools. *School Psychology Review, 23*, 165-174.

Bernstein, J. Y. & Watson, M. W. (1997). Children who are targets of bullying: A victim pattern. *Journal of Interpersonal Violence, 12*, 483-498.

Berthold, K. A. & Hoover, J. H. (2000). Correlates of bullying and victimization among intermediate students in the Midwestern USA. *School Psychology International, 21*, 65-78.

Bosworth, K., Espelage, D. L., & Simon, T. R. (1999). Factors associated with bullying behavior in middle school students. *Journal of Early Adolescence, 19*, 341-362.

Boulton, M. J. & Smith, P. K. (1994). Bully-victim problems in middle-school children: Stability, self-perceived competence, peer perceptions, and peer acceptance. *British Journal of Developmental Psychology, 12*, 315-329.

Craig, W. M. (1998). The relationship among bullying, victimization, depression, anxiety, and aggression in elementary school children. *Personality and Individual Differences, 24*, 123-130.

Dodge, K. A. (1993). Social-cognitive mechanisms in the development of conduct disorder and depression. *Annual Reviews of Psychology, 44*, 559-584.

Dodge, K. & Frame, C. L. (1982). Social cognitive biases and deficits in aggressive boys. *Child Development, 53*, 467-489.

Duncan, R. D. (1999). Maltreatment by parents and peers: The relationship between child abuse, bully victimization, and psychological distress. *Child Maltreatment, 4*, 45-55.

Eslea, M. & Smith, P. (2000). Pupil and parent attitudes towards bullying in primary schools. *European Journal of Psychology of Education, 15*, 207-219.

Espelage, D. L., & Asidao, C. S. (2001). Conversations with middle school students about bullying and victimization: Should we be concerned? *Journal of Emotional Abuse, 2*, 49-62.

Forero, R., McLellan, L., Rissel, C., & Bauman, A. (1999). Bullying behaviour and psychological health among school students in New South Wales, Australia: Cross sectional survey. *British Medical Journal, 319*, 344-348.

Harris, S., Petrie, G., & Willoughby, W. (2002). Bullying among 9th graders: An exploratory study. *NASSP Bulletin, 86,* 3-14.

Haynie, D. L., Nansel, T., Eitel, P., Crump, A. D., Saylor, K., Yu, K., & Simons-Mortons, B. (2001). Bullies, victims, and bully/victims: Distinct groups of at-risk youth. *Journal of Early Adolescence, 21,* 29-49.

Hazler, R. J., Hoover, J. H., & Oliver, R. (1991). Student perceptions of victimization by bullies in school. *Journal of Humanistic Education and Development, 29,* 143-150.

Hoover, J. H., Oliver, R., & Hazler, R. J. (1992). Bullying: Perceptions of adolescent victims in the Midwestern U.S.A. *School Psychology International, 13,* 5-16.

Juvonen, J., Nishina, A., & Graham, S. (2000). Peer harassment, psychological adjustment, and school functioning in early adolescence. *Journal of Educational Psychology, 92,* 349-359.

Kaltiala-Heino, R., Rimpela, M., Marttunen, M., Rimpela, A., & Rantanen, P. (1999). Bullying, depression, and suicidal ideation in Finnish adolescents: School survey. *British Medical Journal, 319,* 348-351.

Kann, L., Kinchen, S. A., Williams B. I., Ross, J. G., Lowry, R., Hill, C. V., Grunbaum, J. A., Blumson, P. S., Collins, J. L., & Kolbe, L. J. (1998). *Youth Risk Behavior Surveillance, 1997.* Atlanta, GA: Centers for Disease Control and Prevention. CDC Surveillance Summaries, August 14, 1998. MMWR; 47 (No. SS-3).

Kumpulainen, K., Rasanen, E., Henttonen, I., Almqvist, F., Kresanov, K., Linna, S., Moilanen, I., Piha, J., Puura, K., & Tamminen, T. (1998). Bullying and psychiatric symptoms among elementary school-age children. *Child Abuse & Neglect, 22,* 705-717.

Limber, S. P., & Small, M. A. (2000, August). *Self-reports of bully-victimization among primary school students.* Paper presented at the annual meeting of the American Psychological Association, Washington, D.C.

Loeber, R., & Dishion, T. J. (1983). Early predictors of male delinquency: A review. *Psychological Bulletin, 94,* 68-99.

Ma, X. (2001). Bullying and being bullied: To what extent are bullies also victims? *American Educational Research Journal, 38,* 351-370.

Menesini, E., Eslea, M., Smith, P. K., Genta, M. L., Giannetti, E., Fonzi, A., & Costebile, A. (1996). Cross-national comparison of children's attitudes towards bully/victim problems in school. *Aggressive Behavior, 23,* 245-257.

Nansel, T. R., Overpeck, M., Pilla, R. S., Ruan, W. J., Simons-Morton, B., & Scheidt, P. (2001). Bullying behaviors among U.S. youth: Prevalence and association with psychosocial adjustment. *Journal of the American Medical Association, 285,* 2094-2100.

Oliver, R., Hoover, J. H., & Hazler, R. J. (1994). The perceived roles of bullying in small-town Midwestern schools. *Journal of Counseling and Development, 72,* 416-420.

Olweus, D. (1978). *Aggression in the schools: Bullies and whipping boys.* New York: Wiley.

Olweus, D. (1993). *Bullying at school: What we know and what we can do.* Oxford, UK: Basil Blackwell.

Pellegrini, A. D. (2001). A longitudinal study of heterosexual relationships, aggression, and sexual harassment during the transition from primary school through middle school. *Applied Developmental Psychology, 22,* 119-133.

Pellegrini, A. D. & Bartini, M. (2000). A longitudinal study of bullying, victimization, and peer affiliation during the transition from primary school to middle school. *American Educational Research Journal, 37,* 699-725.

Pellegrini, A. D., Bartini, M., & Brooks, F. (1999). School bullies, victims, and aggressive victims: Factors relating top group affiliation and victimization in early adolescence. *Journal of Educational Psychology, 91,* 216-224.

Perry, D. G., Kusel, S. J., & Perry, L. C. (1988). Victims of peer aggression. *Developmental Psychology, 24,* 807-814.

Rigby, K. (1997). Attitudes and beliefs about bullying among Australian school children. *Irish Journal of Psychology, 18,* 202-220.

Rigby, K. (1998). The relationship between reported health and involvement in bully/victim problems among male and female secondary schoolchildren. *Journal of Health Psychology, 3,* 465-476.

Rigby, K. (1999). Peer victimization at school and the health of secondary school students. *British Journal of Educational Psychology, 69,* 95-104.

Rigby, K., & Slee, P. T. (1991). Bullying among Australian school children: Reported behavior and attitudes toward victims. *Journal of Social Psychology, 131,* 615-627.

Swearer, S. M. (2001). *The Bully Survey.* Unpublished manuscript, University of Nebraska-Lincoln.

Swearer, S. M. & Doll, B. (2001). Bullying in schools: An ecological framework. *Journal of Emotional Abuse, 2,* 7-23.

Swearer, S. M., Song, S. Y., Cary, P. T., Eagle, J. W., & Mickelson, W. T. (2001). Psychosocial correlates in bullying and victimization: The relationship between depression, anxiety, and bully/victim status. *Journal of Emotional Abuse, 2,* 95-121.

A Cluster Analytic Investigation of Victimization Among High School Students: Are Profiles Differentially Associated with Psychological Symptoms and School Belonging?

Melissa K. Holt

Family Research Laboratory, University of New Hampshire

Dorothy L. Espelage

University of Illinois at Urbana-Champaign

SUMMARY. Victimization experiences of 504 racially diverse high school students were evaluated. Questionnaires assessed sexual harassment victimization, psychological and physical abuse in dating relationships, peer victimization, childhood sexual abuse, school belonging, and psychological functioning. Results showed that 70% of students had been sexually harassed by peers during the past year, 40% had experi-

Address correspondence to: Melissa K. Holt, PhD, Family Research Laboratory, 126 Horton Social Sciences Center, University of New Hampshire, Durham, NH 03824 (E-mail: mkholt@cisunix.unh.edu).

[Haworth co-indexing entry note]: "A Cluster Analytic Investigation of Victimization Among High School Students: Are Profiles Differentially Associated with Psychological Symptoms and School Belonging?" Holt, Melissa K., and Dorothy L. Espelage. Co-published simultaneously in *Journal of Applied School Psychology* (The Haworth Press, Inc.) Vol. 19, No. 2, 2003, pp. 81-98; and: *Bullying, Peer Harassment, and Victimization in the Schools: The Next Generation of Prevention* (ed: Maurice J. Elias, and Joseph E. Zins) The Haworth Press, Inc., 2003, pp. 81-98. Single or multiple copies of this article are available for a fee from The Haworth Document Delivery Service [1-800-HAWORTH, 9:00 a.m. - 5:00 p.m. (EST). E-mail address: docdelivery@haworthpress.com].

http://www.haworthpress.com/store/product.asp?sku=J008
10.1300/J008v19n02_06

enced physical dating violence, 66% had been victimized by emotional abuse in dating relationships, and 54% had been bullied. A cluster analysis of victimization measures revealed heterogeneity in victimization experiences; five distinct groups of students emerged. Individuals who had experienced multiple forms of victimization tended to have lower psychological well-being and a diminished sense of school belonging. Results are discussed in terms of implications for clinical and school interventions. *[Article copies available for a fee from The Haworth Document Delivery Service: 1-800-HAWORTH. E-mail address: <docdelivery@haworthpress.com> Website: <http://www.HaworthPress.com> © 2003 by The Haworth Press, Inc. All rights reserved.]*

KEYWORDS. Adolescence, race, victimization, bullying, harassment

INTRODUCTION

Sexual harassment and dating violence are pervasive forms of victimization within our society. Initial efforts aimed at better understanding these phenomena focused on college students and adults. Results derived from such studies showed that upwards of 50% of women have experienced sexual harassment in their working lives (Fitzgerald & Ormerod, 1993) and as many as 50% have been physically abused by a dating partner (Neufeld, McNamara, & Ertl, 1999). More recently research endeavors have examined the prevalence of sexual harassment and dating violence among adolescents although the literature base for this population is less extensive. Extant literature suggests that it is during adolescence when sexual harassment and dating violence begin to emerge (e.g., American Association of University Women (AAUW), 1993; Burcky, Reuterman, & Kopsky, 1988). Moreover, studies have documented that 80% of high school students have experienced sexual harassment in the form of unwelcome sexual behaviors of a physical and verbal nature (AAUW, 2001). Furthermore, between 10% (Roscoe & Callahan, 1985) and 55% have incurred physical or emotional abuse from a dating partner (O'Keefe, 1998).

The need to understand the dynamics of sexual harassment and dating violence is pressing given the psychological, educational, and career-related outcomes many targets face. For example, individuals who have been sexually harassed often suffer from depression, post-traumatic stress, decreased interest in school- and work-related activities, and self-doubt (AAUW, 1993; Dansky & Kilpatrick, 1997; Schneider, Swan, & Fitzgerald, 1997). Similarly, experiencing dating violence can produce outcomes, including feelings of anger and sadness (Carlson, 1987), post-traumatic stress and anxiety (Harned, 2001). Although some existing research explores sexual harassment and dating violence among adolescents, a comprehensive analysis of how such victimization is linked to psychological functioning is lacking.

Furthermore, additional information is needed regarding the effects of experiencing sexual harassment and dating violence in conjunction with other forms of victimization. Understanding multiple types of victimization affecting an individual is particularly important for two reasons. First, studies have demonstrated that when individuals are victimized once they are at increased risk for future victimization (e.g., Harned, 2000). For example, students who reported experiencing sexual harassment were more likely to report dating violence victimization than those students who had not experienced sexual harassment (Connolly, McMaster, Craig, & Pepler, 1997). Second, victims of multiple types of violence are at greater risk for negative outcomes (e.g., Follette, Polusny, Bechtel, & Naugle, 1996). For instance, college females who had experienced sexual harassment, sexual abuse/assault, and physical abuse reported significantly more post-traumatic stress, anxiety, and disordered eating symptoms than women who had experienced only one type of victimization (Harned, 2000). Given that studies of repeat victimization have focused primarily on college-aged and adult populations, however, we know little about the effects of multiple victimization among adolescents. In the case of middle and high school students a comprehensive model of victimization would be strengthened through the inclusion of peer victimization and childhood sexual abuse in addition to sexual harassment and dating violence.

Peer Victimization

Peer victimization in the form of bullying is a particularly salient factor to consider due to the frequency with which it occurs (Espelage, Bosworth, & Simon, 2000; Hoover, Oliver, & Hazler, 1992). For example, 88% of junior high and high school students reported having observed bullying and 77% reported being a victim of bullying during their school years (Hoover et al., 1992). Although there is substantial variation in how students respond to victimization from their peers (Kochenderfer-Ladd & Ladd, 2001), at least 14% of the Hoover et al. sample reported significant distress as a result of the harassment. Additional research has been directed at understanding why some students experience adverse outcomes to victimization and others do not (Kochenderfer-Ladd & Ladd, 2001). Specifically, these authors postulate that students who lack adaptive coping resources to draw from when they are harassed might experience negative outcomes.

Childhood Sexual Abuse

Childhood sexual abuse is another important form of victimization to evaluate among adolescents for a number of reasons. First, since approximately 20% of females and between 5% and 10% of males experience sexual abuse in childhood or adolescence (Finkelhor, 1994), it is probable that some participants in this investigation have been sexually abused. Second, a childhood sexual abuse history might heighten an individual's likelihood of experiencing subsequent victimization. For example, one study documented that women who had been sexually abused as children were more likely to experience sexual victimization and sexual harassment as adults than women without histories of childhood sexual abuse (Frazier & Cohen, 1992). A similar pattern might exist for adolescents. Third, childhood sexual abuse has been linked to comparable psychological outcomes as those associated with sexual harassment and dating violence, including depression, decreased involvement in school, anxiety, and substance abuse (e.g., Garnefski & Arends, 1998; Luster & Small, 1997; Trickett & McBride-Chang, 1995).

Hypotheses

The high rates of sexual harassment and dating violence among high school students necessitate that further research is conducted within this population to delineate more clearly the dynamics associated with these types of victimization. Moreover, it is essential to consider multiple forms of victimization simultaneously so as to better understand the influence of repeat victimization on psychological and educational functioning. As such, the current investigation evaluated the effects of sexual harassment, dating violence, peer victimization, and childhood sexual abuse on adolescents.

We hypothesized that groups of students would emerge with similar victimization patterns (e.g., no victimization, victimization in multiple realms), and that these groups would differ with respect to psychological functioning and sense of school belonging. Specifically, we predicted that on average students in groups characterized by greater victimization would report more symptoms of psychological distress and a lower sense of school belonging than students in groups characterized by less victimization.

The current investigation adds to existing literature by providing a unique perspective on victimization among adolescents. Findings are essential for school employees and clinicians who work with adolescents. Results provide school personnel with a framework for understanding that the victimization experiences of students are heterogeneous and as such victimization might differentially affect students.

METHOD

Participants

Participants were 504 students (grades nine through twelve) from the sole high school in a Midwestern town nearby a large university community. Total enrollment at this school was 1,555. Students enrolled in physical education classes were targeted; given enrollment characteristics of these classes each grade was not proportionally represented although on other demographic characteristics participants were representative of the school population. One hundred eighty-eight participants were Freshmen (37%), 35 were Sophomores (7%), 158 were Juniors (31%), 119 were Seniors (24%), and 4 did not report their grades (< 1%). The mean age for the sample was 16 ($SD = 1.3$). There were 228 (45%) males, 273 (54%) females, and 3 (< 1%) students who did not report their gender. With respect to race there were 131 African-American (26%), 313 Caucasian (62%), 29 Hispanic (6%), 6 Asian-American (1%), 5 Native American (1%), 18 "Other" (4%), and two students (< 1%) who did not report their race.

Procedure

Parental consent. Passive parental consent was used in this investigation to maximize participation. Parents of all students enrolled in physical education classes were sent letters informing them about the purpose of the study. Furthermore, parents were asked to sign the form and return it only if they were unwilling to have their child participate in the investigation; no forms were returned. In addition to passive parental consent, students were asked to consent to participate in the study through an informed consent form included in the questionnaire packet.

Survey administration. Six trained research assistants, the primary researcher, and a faculty member collected data. At least two of these individuals administered surveys to each physical education class, which ranged in size from 25 to 50. Students were first informed about the general nature of the investigation. Next, researchers made certain that students were sitting far enough from one another to ensure confidentiality. Students were then given survey packets and asked to answer all questions honestly, and were told that no identifying information would be associated with their responses. Researchers were available to answer questions that emerged once students began responding to survey items. When students had completed the surveys they were given the opportunity to have their data removed from analyses if they had not carefully considered each question. Each participant was also provided with a list of phone numbers to call (e.g., community counseling agencies) should they experience an emotional reaction to the questionnaires. Last, a raffle was held in each group in which one student won a $10 gift certificate to a local mall. On average it took students approximately 45 minutes to complete the survey.

Measures

Each participant first completed a demographic questionnaire that included questions about his/her sex, age, grade, and race. For race, participants were given six options: African-American (not Hispanic), Asian-American, White (not Hispanic), Hispanic, Native American, and Other (with a space to write in the most appropriate racial descriptor).

Peer sexual harassment. The AAUW Sexual Harassment Survey (AAUW, 1993) is a 14-item inventory designed to measure the frequency with which students are victimized by sexually harassing behaviors. Participants are asked to indicate how often other students engaged in particular behaviors aimed at the participant (e.g., made sexual comments, jokes, gestures, or looks) within the previous year. Items reflect verbal and physical harassment. Response options are: Not sure, Never, Rarely, Occasionally, and Often. Coefficient alpha for this sample was .90 for peers.

Physical victimization in dating relationships. The Victimization in Dating Relationships scale (Foshee et al., 1996) is an 18-item inventory designed to measure physically violent victimization within dating relationships. Participants are asked to indicate how often individuals they went on dates with engaged in particular behaviors (e.g., scratched me, kicked me) and are instructed to count only behaviors that their partners inflicted on them first. Violence inflicted due to self-defense, therefore, is not measured by the Victimization in Dating Relationships scale. There are four response options: Never, 1 to 3 times, 4 to 9 times, and 10 or more times. For the current sample the coefficient alpha was .95.

Psychological abuse in dating relationships. The Abusive Behavior Inventory (ABI; Shepard & Campbell, 1992) is a 30-item inventory designed to measure participants' perceptions of physical and psychological abuse in dating relationships. For the purpose of this investigation, a modified version of the ABI was used. Specifically, 10 items tapping psychological abuse (e.g., "How often has a dating partner called you a name and/or criticized you?") were selected on the basis of appropriateness for a high school sample. Response options offered ranged from 0 (Never) to 4 (Often), and participants were also given the opportunity to select 'Not sure' as a response. The resulting alpha coefficient for the current study was .90.

Peer victimization. A four-item victimization scale was used to assess peer victimization (Espelage & Holt, 2001). This scale was developed through in-depth interviews with middle-school students, emerged as a distinct dimension in a factor analysis of 422 middle school students, and converged with peer nomination data (Espelage & Holt, 2001). Students are asked how often they have been picked on, made fun of, called names, and hit or pushed in the last 30 days. Response options are 'Never,' '1 or 2 times,' '3 or 4 times,' '5 to 6 times,' and '7 or more times.' Coefficient alpha in this sample was .85.

Childhood sexual abuse. The 7-item sexual abuse scale from the Childhood Trauma Questionnaire was used (CTQ; Bernstein et al., 1994). Items on the scale inquire specifically about sexual abuse (e.g., "Someone molested me") and ask about behaviors consistent with sexual abuse (e.g., "Someone tried to make me do sexual things or watch sexual things"). Respondents were asked to think about how often these behaviors occurred throughout their entire lives. Response options are 'Never true,' 'Rarely true,' 'Sometimes true,' 'Often true,' and 'Very often true.' Coefficient alpha for the sexual abuse scale was .85 in this sample.

Psychological functioning. The anxiety/depression scale from the Youth Self-Report (YRS; Achenbach, 1991) was used to assess psychological functioning. This scale consists of 16 self-report items and students are asked to indicate the degree to which particular statements apply to them (e.g., 'I feel lonely,' 'I am nervous or tense'). Response options are 'Not true,' 'Somewhat or sometimes true,' and 'Very true or Often true.' For the current investigation coefficient alpha was .90.

Two scales from the Weinberger Adjustment Inventory's (WAI; Weinberger & Schwartz, 1990) Psychological Distress Scale were also used, self-esteem and low well-being. Response options are on a 5-point scale ranging from 'not at all true' through 'always true.' For the current sample, coefficient alpha was .77.

Sense of school belonging. Perceived belonging at school was assessed with a revised version of the Psychological Sense of School Membership scale (Goodenow, 1993). This scale was a result of a factor analysis based on 558 middle-school students; for a more detailed description of the development refer to Bosworth et al. (1999). Students are asked how much they agree with the following statements: 'I feel proud of belonging to my school,' 'I am treated with as much respect as other students are,' 'The teachers here respect me,' and 'There is at least one teacher or other adult in this school I can talk to if I have a problem.' Response options include 'Strongly disagree,' 'Disagree,' 'Neither agree nor disagree,' 'Agree,' and 'Strongly agree.' Coefficient alpha for the current sample was .66.

RESULTS

First, frequencies of victimization were computed. Analyses indicated that 70% of the adolescents surveyed had experienced peer sexual harassment at least 'rarely' and 54% had experienced peer sexual harassment at least 'occasionally' within the last year. With respect to dating violence, 66% of the students endorsed psychological abuse in dating relationships and 40% reported incurring physical violence from a dating partner. Finally, 54% of respondents noted that they had been bullied during the last 30 days. Frequencies by gender and grade are delineated in Table 1.

Second, correlations among study variables were examined. As delineated in Table 2, for males and females victimization variables were positively correlated with one another, with correlations ranging from low to moderate in strength. In addition, victimization was related to psychological functioning; greater victimization tended to be associated with greater psychological distress. Finally, a diminished sense of school belonging was positively correlated with victimization and psychological symptoms.

Third, we used cluster analytic techniques to identify types of victimization profiles yielded by high school students. The following scales were entered into the SYSTAT program using a *k*-means cluster analytic procedure: peer sexual harassment, physical dating violence, psychological abuse in dating relationships, peer victimization, and childhood sexual abuse. Sufficient scale data were available for 491 participants. Results of cluster analyses utilizing these methods suggested that a five-cluster solution was appropriate for the data (see Table 3).

Designated labels for each cluster were: (1) 'No victimization' (Cluster 1), a group characterized by scores below the mean on all victimization measures; (2) 'Sexual harassment' (Cluster 2), a group characterized by scores one standard deviation above the mean on peer sexual harassment and scores within one standard deviation of the mean on all other victimization indicators; (3) 'Re-victimization' (Cluster 3), a group characterized by scores one standard deviation above the mean on all victimization measures *except* peer victimization; (4) 'Psychological abuse in dating relationships' (Cluster 4), a group characterized by scores one standard deviation above the mean on psychological abuse in dating relationships and scores within one standard deviation of the mean on all other victimization measures; (5) 'Physical dating violence and childhood sexual abuse' (Cluster 5), a group characterized by scores three standard deviations above the mean on physical dating violence, one standard deviation above the mean on childhood sexual abuse, and within one standard deviation of the mean on all other victimization measures.

TABLE 1. Victimization Frequencies by Grade and Gender

	Total Sample		Grade 9		Grade 10		Grade 11		Grade 12	
	M (N = 228)	F (N = 273)	M (N = 83)	F (N = 105)	M (N = 22)	F (N = 13)	M (N = 70)	F (N = 87)	M (N = 52)	F (N = 66)
Peer sexual harassment										
Rarely	60%	75%	52%	71%	60%	85%	60%	75%	69%	79%
Occasionally	42%	54%	31%	49%	46%	69%	41%	56%	56%	56%
Physical abuse in dating relationships	43%	41%	34%	33%	50%	61%	39%	52%	50%	38%
Emotional abuse in dating relationships	59%	71%	46%	71%	64%	92%	59%	79%	77%	71%
Peer victimization	57%	52%	48%	50%	50%	62%	70%	52%	58%	56%

TABLE 2. Correlations Among Study Variables by Gender

	CSA	DV	PA	PSH	PV	LSE	LWB	Anx/Dep	Belong
CSA		0.40**	0.25**	0.22**	0.06	0.08	0.06	0.37**	−0.23**
DV	0.45**		0.39**	0.32**	0.14*	0.23**	0.18**	0.48**	−0.20**
PA	0.36**	0.65**		0.33**	0.07	0.19**	0.11	0.31**	−0.24**
PSH	0.51**	0.42**	0.43**		0.00	−0.03	−0.03	0.10	−0.16*
PV	0.20**	0.12*	0.27**	0.22**		0.18**	0.10	0.26**	−0.06
LSE	0.18**	0.22**	0.30**	0.17**	0.20**		0.56**	0.57**	−0.32**
LWB	0.17**	0.22**	0.28**	0.17**	0.15*	0.55**		0.49**	−0.24**
Anx/Dep	0.35**	0.34**	0.40**	0.28**	0.33**	0.61**	0.50**		−0.30**
Belong	−0.09	−0.11	−0.17**	−0.10	−0.03	−0.25**	−0.25**	−0.13*	

Note. Upper right quadrant represents males and lower right quadrant represents females. * $p < .05$. ** $p < .01$. CSA = Childhood sexual abuse from Childhood Trauma Questionnaire; DV = Physical dating violence from the Victimization in Relationships Scale; PA = Psychological abuse in dating relationships from the Abusive Behavior Inventory; PSH = Peer sexual harassment from the AAUW Sexual Harassment Inventory; PV = Peer victimization from the Self-reported Victimization Scale; LSE = Low self-esteem scale from the Weinberger Adjustment Inventory; LWB = Low well-being scale from the Weinberger Adjustment Inventory; Anx/Dep = Anxiety/Depression scale from the Youth Self Report; Belong = Sense of School Belonging from Psychological Sense of School Membership Scale.

Chi-square analyses revealed that these clusters did not differ by grade or race, but that they did differ by gender (χ^2 (1, $N = 493$) = 12.69, $p < .01$). Specifically, a greater percentage of females were in the 'Psychological abuse in dating relationships' cluster than males, and a greater percentage of males were in the 'Physical dating violence and childhood sexual abuse' cluster than females.

Next, we evaluated the extent to which the cluster groups differed on psychological symptoms, including sense of school belonging, depression/anxiety scores from the Youth Self-Report (Achenbach, 1991) and psychological low well-being and self-esteem scores from the Weinberger Adjustment Inventory (Weinberger & Schwartz, 1990). Given that these variables were correlated moderately with one another we conducted a MANOVA with cluster membership as the independent variable and school belonging, anxiety/depression, low well-being, and self-esteem as dependent variables. A significant group difference emerged from this analysis (Wilks's lambda = .75, F = 9.16, $p < .05$, eta-squared = .07). Follow-up univariate tests indicated that there was a significant group difference for each of the seven dependent variables (Fs = 4.70-31.27, $ps < .01$; see Table 3).

A number of key findings emerged. Not surprisingly, the 'No victimization' cluster group had lower scores on psychological distress than the remaining four cluster groups. In addition, the 'Re-victimization' group reported a significantly lower sense of school belonging than the 'Peer sexual harassment' and 'Psychological abuse in dating relationships' groups and lower self-esteem than the other four groups. Moreover, members of the 'Re-victimization' group revealed significantly more depression and lower well-being than individuals in the 'No Victimization' and 'Peer sexual harassment' groups, and more anxiety/depression than individuals in all groups except for the 'Physical dating violence and childhood sexual abuse' group.

Finally, to determine which psychological variable was the most predictive of cluster membership, a discriminant function analysis (DFA) was calculated. Only one discriminant function was statistically significant (Wilks's lambda = .75, χ^2 = 140.42, $p < .001$). Interpretation of the structure coefficients indicated that the Depression/Anxiety (.92) had the highest correlation with the discriminant function, followed by low self-esteem (.52), school belonging ($-.47$), and low well-being (.35). This is consistent with the effect size data presented in Table 4. Although the small sample sizes in the cluster groups prohibit additional analyses, these results suggest that anxiety and depression significantly differentiates several of the groups, particularly clusters 3 and 5.

TABLE 3. Means and Standard Deviations for Each Victimization Scale Across Clusters

SCALE	Total Sample[a]		'No victimization' (Cluster 1[b])		'Peer sexual harassment' (Cluster 2[c])		'Re-victimization' (Cluster 3[d])		'Psychological abuse in dating relationships' (Cluster 4[e])		'Physical dating violence and childhood sexual abuse' (Cluster 5[f])	
	M	SD	M	SD	M	SD	M	SD	M	SD	M	SD
Childhood sexual abuse	7.59	4.28	6.36	3.13	8.94	4.23	15.58	5.10	7.68	4.10	13.06	5.24
Psychological abuse in dating relationships	5.22	6.13	1.84	2.34	5.60	4.34	17.21	7.15	13.37	4.54	8.78	6.54
Physical dating violence	3.28	7.33	0.48	1.36	2.21	2.72	19.05	10.34	4.83	5.01	27.72	11.08
Peer sexual harassment	5.78	7.53	1.82	2.24	14.68	5.37	27.68	7.61	5.29	4.10	12.94	6.76
Peer victimization	6.26	3.42	5.76	2.93	6.65	3.93	7.26	4.15	6.85	3.66	9.06	4.61

Note. [a]n = 491, [b]n = 295, [c]n = 72, [d]n = 22, [e]n = 82, [f]n = 20.

TABLE 4. Means and Standard Deviations for Sense of School Belonging and Psychological Symptoms Across Clusters

	Total Sample[a]		'No victimization' (Cluster 1[b])		'Peer sexual harassment' (Cluster 2[c])		'Re-victimization' (Cluster 3[d])		'Psychological abuse in dating relationships' (Cluster 4[e])		'Physical dating violence and childhood sexual abuse' (Cluster 5[f])		F	Eta-Squared
	M	SD	M	SD	M	SD	M	SD	M	SD	M	SD		
School Belonging	14.63	3.24	15.19	2.84	14.34	3.54	12.14	4.59	13.91	3.16	13.05	3.37	8.32*	.06
Low Self-Esteem	13.73	5.62	12.65	5.02	14.10	5.85	19.23	4.93	15.54	6.50	14.95	4.56	11.62*	.09
Low Well-Being	13.53	5.83	12.76	5.43	13.88	6.19	16.90	7.02	14.57	6.32	15.55	4.50	4.70*	.04
Anxiety/Depression	6.56	6.63	4.68	5.12	6.72	6.43	15.50	8.00	8.95	6.76	14.10	8.13	31.27*	.21

Note. [a] $n = 491$, [b] $n = 295$, [c] $n = 72$, [d] $n = 22$, [e] $n = 82$, [f] $n = 20$. * $p < .01$. School Belonging from the Psychological Sense of School Membership Scale; Low Self-Esteem from the Weinberger Adjustment Inventory; Low Well-Being from the Weinberger Adjustment Inventory; Anxiety/Depression from the Youth Self-Report.

DISCUSSION

The current investigation examined sexual harassment, dating violence, peer victimization, and childhood sexual abuse among racially diverse adolescents. Objectives were (1) to gain a better understanding of prevalence rates, and (2) to delineate psychological and educational effects of victimization patterns.

Results indicated that adolescents from the high school surveyed incur frequent victimization across multiple realms. Within this sample, 70% of the participants reported that they had been sexually harassed by peers. This rate is similar to those cited in previous studies. For example, in the AAUW (1993) sample 79% of the adolescents surveyed endorsed peer sexual harassment. With respect to dating violence, 40% of the respondents in this investigation indicated that they had been physically abused by a dating partner and 66% revealed that they had experienced emotional abuse from a dating partner. These rates are also consistent with existing literature (e.g., Bookwala et al., 1992; Roscoe & Callahan, 1985). Finally, in line with past research (Nansel et al., 2001), 54% of the high school students in this study noted that they had been victimized by peers within the last month.

Findings also supported the hypothesis that there is heterogeneity in victimization experiences among these high school students. Five distinct groups of students with similar victimization histories were identified using cluster analysis. These groups included (1) students with minimal victimization experiences, (2) adolescents who reported only significant peer sexual harassment, (3) participants who revealed only significant psychological abuse in dating relationships, (4) respondents with significant physical dating violence and childhood sexual abuse experiences, and (5) a small number of adolescents who reported experiencing multiple forms of victimization. As such, our findings suggested that while some students are victimized in primarily one realm (e.g., they are sexually harassed), other adolescents are the targets of multiple types of victimization. This supports limited existing literature that sexual harassment and dating violence in particular are likely to co-occur (e.g., Connolly et al., 1997).

Interestingly, resulting clusters did not differ by grade or race, but did differ by gender. In support of previous literature indicating that females experience more psychological abuse in dating relationships than males (e.g., Foshee, 1996), girls in this sample were more likely than boys to be classified in the group characterized by high levels of psychological abuse in dating relationships. Surprisingly, males were somewhat more likely than females to be members of the 'Physical dating violence and Childhood sexual abuse' group; this counters previous literature finding that either gender differences on physical dating violence did not exist (e.g., Malik, Sorenson, & Aneshensel, 1997) or females were more often the targets of physical dating violence than males (e.g., Roscoe & Callahan, 1985).

As expected, victimization patterns were differentially related to psychological functioning and sense of school belonging. For instance, members of the 'No victimization' group were less distressed than individuals in the other four groups, suggesting that being the target of even one type of victimization produces deleterious psychological symptoms. Consistent with hypotheses, negative outcomes were heightened, however, for adolescents in the 'Re-victimization' group. Importantly, not only did these adolescents reveal more psychological symptoms (e.g., more depression) than individuals in some of the other groups, but they also reported feeling disconnected to the school environment. These findings support the notion advocated by Follette and colleagues (1996) that individuals who are re-victimized tend to suffer more distress. Coupled together these risk factors might result in students disengaging in school activities or dropping out. As such, it is critical to identify students who might have multiple victimization experiences to provide support structures for them.

Limitations of the Study

Future studies are needed to replicate findings from the current investigation and to further our understanding of multiple victimization among adolescents. Results from the present study are limited to a suburban population and, therefore, might not be applicable to urban youth. Furthermore, a restricted range of outcomes was considered; the effects of victimization on areas such as academic performance and social functioning with peers and family are also important to evaluate. Finally, this investigation was cross-sectional in nature and, therefore, it was impossible to discern whether students with multiple victimization experiences had changes in functioning after they first were victimized or whether changes occurred as a result of cumulative effects.

Implications for Research and Practice in Applied Psychology

In sum, individuals are faced with multiple forms of victimization during their high school years, including sexual harassment, dating violence, peer victimization, and childhood sexual abuse. These experiences are not to be taken lightly; adolescents are negatively affected when they are targets of such victimization. Furthermore, although school personnel might believe that girls are victimized more frequently than males, this study documents that males are also frequently targets. In particular, it appears that males are more likely than females to report a combination of physical dating violence and childhood sexual abuse.

Findings from the current investigation also underscore the importance of understanding adolescents' overall victimization experiences rather than considering specific types in isolation from one another. Similarly, results highlight the salience of addressing a range of victimization types in educational or intervention programming. Furthermore, school psychologists should be aware that students presenting with one victimization concern might also have been victimized in additional arenas.

Given the developmental importance of adolescence it is possible that psychological distress resulting from victimization will have deleterious effects on myriad aspects of these individuals' lives as they transition into adulthood. It is, therefore, incumbent upon researchers and educators to promote awareness of these issues, and to create environments that feel safe enough for high school students to approach school staff to obtain help in curbing violent behaviors directed toward them and to seek psychological counseling if necessary.

REFERENCES

Achenbach, T.M. (1991). *Manual for the Youth Self-Report and 1991 Profile.*

American Association of University Women Educational Foundation (2001). *Hostile hallways: Sexual harassment and bullying in schools.* Washington, DC: Harris/Scholastic Research.

American Association of University Women Educational Foundation (1993). *Hostile hallways: The AAUW survey on sexual harassment in America's schools* (Research Report 923012). Washington, DC: Harris/Scholastic Research.

Bernstein, D.P., & Fink, L. (1998). *Childhood Trauma Questionnaire: A Retrospective Self-Report Manual.* San Antonio: The Psychological Corporation.

Bookwala, J., Frieze, I.H., Smith, C., & Ryan, K. (1992). Predictors of dating violence: A multivariate analysis. *Violence and Victims, 7,* 297-309.

Bosworth, K., Espelage, D.L., & Simon, T. (1999). Factors associated with bullying behavior in middle school students. *Journal of Early Adolescence, 19,* 341-362.

Burcky, W., Reuterman, N., & Kopsky, S. (1988). Dating violence among high school students. *The School Counselor, 35,* 353-358.

Carlson, B.E. (1987). Dating violence: A research review and comparison with spouse abuse. *Social Casework: The Journal of Contemporary Social Work,* 16-23.

Connolly, J., McMaster, L., Craig, W., & Pepler, D. (1997). Dating, puberty, and sexualized aggression. In A. Slep (Chair), *Dating Violence: Predictors and Consequences in Normative and At-Risk Populations.* Symposium conducted at the annual meeting of the Association for the Advancement of Behavior Therapy, Miami, FL.

Dansky, B.S., & Kilpatrick, D.G. (1997). Effects of sexual harassment. In W.T. O'Donohue (Ed.), *Sexual harassment: Theory, research, and treatment* (pp. 152-174). Needham Heights, MA: Allyn & Bacon.

Espelage, D.L., Bosworth, K., & Simon, T. (2000). Examining the social environment of middle school students who bully. *Journal of Counseling and Development, 78,* 326-333.

Espelage, D.L., & Holt, M.K. (2001). Bullying and victimization during early adolescence: Peer influences and psychosocial correlates. *Journal of Emotional Abuse, 2 (3),* 123-142.

Finkelhor, D. (1994) Current information on the scope and nature of child sexual abuse. *Future of Children, 4,* 31-53.

Fitzgerald, L.F., & Ormerod, A.J. (1993). Breaking the silence: The sexual harassment of women in academia and the workplace. In F.L. Denmark & M.A. Paludi (Eds.), *Psychology of women: A handbook of issues and theories* (pp. 553-581). Westport, CT: Greenwood Press/Greenwood Publishing Group, Inc.

Follette, V.M., Polusny, M.A., Bechtle, A.E., & Naugle, A.E. (1996). Cumulative trauma: The impact of child sexual abuse, adult sexual assault, and spouse abuse. *Journal of Traumatic Stress, 9,* 25-35.

Foshee, V.A. (1996). Gender differences in adolescent dating abuse prevalence, types, and injuries. *Health Education Research: Theory and Practice, 11,* 275-286.

Foshee, V.A., Linder, G.F., Bauman, C.E., & Langwick, S.A. (1996). The safe dates project: Theoretical basis, evaluation, design, and selected baseline findings. *American Journal of Preventive Medicine, 12,* 39-47.

Frazier, P.A., & Cohen, B.B. (1992). Research on the sexual victimization of women: Implications for counselor training. *The Counseling Psychologist, 20,* 141-158.

Garnefski, N., & Arends, E. (1998). Sexual abuse and adolescent maladjustment: Differences between male and female victims. *Journal of Adolescence, 21,* 99-107.

Goodenow, C. (1993). The psychological sense of school membership among adolescents: Scale development and educational correlates. *Psychology in the Schools, 30,* 79-90.

Harned, M. (2001). Abused women or abused men? An examination of the context and outcomes of dating abuse. *Violence and Victims, 16,* 269-285.

Harned, M.S. (2000, May). *The extent and impact of repeated and multiple victimization.* Paper presented at the 72nd Annual Meeting of the Midwestern Psychological Association, Chicago, IL.

Hoover, J.H., Oliver, R., & Hazler, R.J. (1992). Bullying: Perceptions of adolescent victims in the midwestern USA. *School Psychology International, 13,* 5-16.

Kochenderfer-Ladd, B., & Ladd, G.W. (2001). Variations in peer victimization: Relations to children's maladjustment. In J. Juvonen & S. Graham (Eds.), *Peer harassment in school: The plight of the vulnerable and victimized* (pp. 25-48). New York: Guilford Press.

Luster, T., & Small, S.A. (1997). Sexual abuse history and problems in adolescence: Exploring the effects of moderating variables. *Journal of Marriage and the Family, 59,* 131-142.

Malik, S., Sorenson, S.B., & Aneshensel, C.S. (1997). Community and dating violence among adolescents: Perpetration and victimization. *Journal of Adolescent Health, 21*, 291-302.

Nansel, T.R., Overpeck, M., Pilla, R.S., Ruan, W. J., Simons-Morton, B., & Scheidt, P. (2001). Bullying behaviors among US youth: Prevalence and association with psychosocial adjustment. *Journal of the American Medical Association, 285*, 2094-2132.

Neufeld, J., McNamara, J.R., & Ertl, M. (1999). Incidence and prevalence of dating partner abuse and its relation to dating practices. *Journal of Interpersonal Violence, 14*, 125-137.

O'Keefe, M. (1998). Factors mediating the link between witnessing interparental violence and dating violence. *Journal of Family Violence, 13*, 39-57.

Roscoe, B., & Callahan, J.E. (1985). Adolescents' self-report of violence in families and dating relations. *Adolescence, 20*, 1985.

Schneider, K.T., Swan, S., & Fitzgerald, L.F. (1997). Job-related psychological effects of sexual harassment in the workplace: Empirical evidence from two organizations. *Journal of Applied Psychology, 82*, 401-415.

Shepard, M.F., & Campbell, J.A. (1992). The Abusive Behavior Inventory: A measure of psychological and physical abuse. *Journal of Interpersonal Violence, 7*, 291-305.

Trickett, P.K., & McBride-Chang, C. (1995). The developmental impact of different forms of child abuse and neglect. *Developmental Review, 15*, 311-337.

Weinberger, D.A., & Schwartz, G.E. (1990). Distress and restraint as superordinate dimensions of self-reported adjustment: A typological perspective. *Journal of Personality, 58*, 381-417.

Immigrant Children in Austria: Aggressive Behavior and Friendship Patterns in Multicultural School Classes

Dagmar Strohmeier
Christiane Spiel

University of Vienna, Austria

SUMMARY. As a consequence of worldwide waves of immigration there is a permanent increase of ethnically mixed school classes in countries all over the world. However, there is a lack of empirical studies on interethnic relationships which differentiate immigrant children based on their countries of origin. The present paper focuses on these topics and provides data of both negative and positive aspects of interethnic interactions. Direct and indirect forms of bullying, friendship patterns, and peer acceptance in 326 native and 242 immigrant children aged 11 to 14 (57% native Austrian, 22% former Yugoslavian, 14% Turkish/Kurdish,

Address correspondence to: Dagmar Strohmeier, University of Vienna, Department of Psychology, Center for Educational Psychology & Evaluation, Universitätsstraße 7, A-1010 Wien (E-mail: dagmar.strohmeier@univie.ac.at).

The authors are grateful to all the schools, teachers and pupils who participated in this study.

Parts of this paper were presented at the 5th workshop on aggression in Hannover, Germany, November, 2000.

[Haworth co-indexing entry note]: "Immigrant Children in Austria: Aggressive Behavior and Friendship Patterns in Multicultural School Classes." Strohmeier, Dagmar, and Christiane Spiel. Co-published simultaneously in *Journal of Applied School Psychology* (The Haworth Press, Inc.) Vol. 19, No. 2, 2003, pp. 99-116; and: *Bullying, Peer Harassment, and Victimization in the Schools: The Next Generation of Prevention* (ed: Maurice J. Elias, and Joseph E. Zins) The Haworth Press, Inc., 2003, pp. 99-116. Single or multiple copies of this article are available for a fee from The Haworth Document Delivery Service [1-800-HAWORTH, 9:00 a.m. - 5:00 p.m. (EST). E-mail address: docdelivery@haworthpress.com].

http://www.haworthpress.com/store/product.asp?sku=J008
© 2003 by The Haworth Press, Inc. All rights reserved.
10.1300/J008v19n02_07

7% rest group) in 29 ethnically mixed school classes (6th and 7th grades) were examined. Bullying was measured via the Olweus Bully/Victim Questionnaire and via peer nomination techniques, friendship patterns via self-ratings. Peer acceptance was defined by social preference scores on positive and negative sociometric items. According to peer ratings Austrian children were found to be more often victims (9%) and bullies (12%) of direct bullying than immigrant children. Prevalence rates in immigrant children varied depending on their country of origin between 2% and 8% for victims and 3% to 7% for bullies. Results suggested that Turkish/Kurdish children are at risk concerning their social integration in class (e.g., they had the fewest number of friends in class, reported higher levels of loneliness at school, and were less accepted by their peers compared to Austrians and former Yugoslavian children). Friendship patterns differed considerably between native children and children of the three immigrant groups. Findings are discussed concerning differences in integration strategies of immigrant children depending on their country of origin. *[Article copies available for a fee from The Haworth Document Delivery Service: 1-800-HAWORTH. E-mail address: <docdelivery@haworthpress.com> Website: <http://www.HaworthPress.com> © 2003 by The Haworth Press, Inc. All rights reserved.]*

KEYWORDS. Immigrant children, interethnic interactions, bullying, peer acceptance, friendship, integration strategies

As a consequence of worldwide waves of immigration, a growing number of immigrant children are attending public schools together with native borns in countries all over the world. This development leads to an increase of ethnically mixed school classes. There, children are challenged to learn cooperative forms of interethnic interactions by crossing cultural group boundaries.

At the moment, scientific knowledge about the quality of interethnic relationships in children is very limited, because the main focus of research lay on prejudices and interethnic attitudes. Interethnic relationships in contact situations were hardly ever studied (e.g., Vedder & O'Dowd, 1999). The present study deals with this topic. To get insights in quality of relationships between immigrant and native children, positive and negative aspects of interactions in multicultural school classes were investigated. Thus, the brief review of the literature incorporates two fields of research: (1) research on aggression, in particular on bullying, and (2) research on friendship, both with the focus on interethnic interactions.

PROBLEMATIC INTERETHNIC INTERACTIONS– PEER AGGRESSION

In the literature dealing with multicultural school classes, one important factor for the formation and maintenance of interactions between pupils from various cultural backgrounds was seen in the proficiency in a common language (Vedder & O'Dowd, 1999). It was argued that a lack of common language skills might hamper the contact between pupils and might be a reason for problematic interethnic relationships in children. To test this hypothesis, Vedder and O'Dowd (1999) conducted a study in ethnically mixed school classes in Sweden. Immigrant children divided into two groups depending on their proficiency in Swedish and Swedish children were compared in peer-rated aggressive-disruptive behavior, isolation/withdrawal and sociability/leadership. No differences between the three groups were found in aggressiveness and withdrawal. However, immigrant children with weaker Swedish comprehension were found to score lower in leadership/sociability compared to their Swedish peers. The importance of good language proficiency for high social status is not limited to immigrant children. In a sociometric study, Rost and Czeschlik (1994) showed the general importance of good verbal comprehension for high social status. Even in monocultural settings, children with higher verbal ability are more accepted by their peers than others. These findings support the impact of language proficiency on peer acceptance but not on negative aspects of interethnic relationships such as aggression.

In general, scientific knowledge concerning immigrant children's involvement in peer aggression is very limited. Only a few studies provide data of prevalence rates. However, these studies never distinguished between the countries of origin of the children (they were uniformly labeled as "foreigners") and did not reveal consistent results. While Fuchs (1999) observed a higher level of aggression in immigrant children than in native born children, some studies revealed no significant differences (Loesel, Bliesener, & Averbeck, 1999; Popp, 2000). In the study conducted by Klicpera and Gasteiger-Klicpera (1996) immigrant children were shown to be less often engaged in bullying than native borns. However, it was argued (e.g., Fuchs, 1999; Popp, 2000) that immigrant children are more likely to attend schools with generally high aggression rates and thus, comparisons of children with different nationalities without controlling for school might be biased. These inconsistencies may also trace back to conceptual differences between the studies concerning peer aggression or to the heterogeneity within the sample of "foreign" children investigated.

The literature on peer aggression shows a high variability in the conceptualization of aggression and the categorization of negative acts. In the last decade more and more empirical studies conducted in schools are based on the concept of bullying according to Olweus (1993) which describes a subcategory of aggression. In this concept a specific relationship between a victim and its perpetrator(s) is defined. The main characteristics of this harmful relationship are imbalance of power, long duration, and the bully's intention to hurt the victim. Bullying is a widespread phenomenon in schools which takes place in almost every schoolclass (Schuster, 1999; Strohmeier & Spiel, 2001). Bullying is also considered as a social phenomenon determined not only by characteristics of bullies and victims but also by social relationships in the group, which were studied between pupils taking different roles (e.g., Salmivalli, Lagerspetz, Bjoerqvist, & Oestermann, 1996; Sutton & Smith, 1999). Furthermore, bullying includes a variety of negative acts which can be delivered face-to-face or by indirect means. Whereas physical or verbal insults are mostly visible and thus categorized as direct bullying, in the last decade various forms of indirect aggressive acts have gained attention (Lagerspetz, Bjoerqvist, & Peltonen, 1988; Bjoerqvist, Lagerspetz, & Kaukiainen, 1992). While Olweus (1993) defines indirect aggression as social exclusion, Lagerspetz et al. (1988, 1992) suggest social manipulation as the main characteristic of indirect bullying. Recently, social manipulative forms of aggression were intensely investigated and found to be typical for girls (e.g., Crick & Grotpeter, 1995; Lagerspetz & Bjoerqvist, 1994; Rys & Bear, 1997). Due to the fact that both gender and race segregation is quite prevalent in children's social lives (Maccoby, 1988, 1990), social exclusion might be more typical for interethnic relationships than social manipulation. Thus, in the present study indirect aggression was defined in terms of social exclusion (Olweus, 1989, 1993).

Cooperative Forms of Interethnic Interactions–Friendships

Scientific knowledge about cooperative forms of interethnic relationships in children is also very limited. However, gender and race were found to be important dimensions along which children form peer groups and dyadic friendships (e.g., Brown, 1990; Boulton & Smith, 1996; Graham & Cohen, 1997). Brown (1995) noted that children are usually able to discriminate between in-group and out-group members at the age of three years. Here, gender appeared to be a more salient factor than race for children's friendship choices (Graham, Cohen, Zbikowski, & Secrist, 1998). The proportion of same gender and same race relationships increases with age (Graham et al., 1998; Maharaj & Connolly, 1994). That means, children exist in different subcultures which are determined by social categories, especially by gender (Maccoby, 1988, 1990). Moreover, the similarity-attraction hypothesis (Berscheid, 1985) could be confirmed for children. Children were shown to be similar to their friends with respect to demographic, behavioral and academic attributes (e.g., Kupersmidt, DeRosier, & Patterson, 1995). Furthermore, the absence of cooperative forms of social relationships is strongly associated with the concept of indirect bullying according to Olweus (1989, 1993) as social exclusion is the defining criterion.

Although the development and maintenance of social relations with members of other cultural groups is a major dimension in acculturation models (e.g., Berry, 1980; Douilis, Moïse, Perréault, & Seneca, 1997), neither interethnic friendship patterns nor peer acceptance were yet investigated in children from different countries of origin. This lack of research is hard to understand, as the formation of close interpersonal relationships is considered an important factor for the social integration of an individual into the peer group (Laireiter & Baumann, 1992).

It is the main goal of the present study to overcome these deficiencies in the research on immigrant children and (1) to distinguish immigrants with respect to their countries of origin, and (2) to focus on both problematic interethnic interactions and cooperative forms of interethnic interactions. Concretely, we addressed the following questions:

- Do children of various immigrant groups (e.g., Turkish, Yugoslavian) differ from each other with respect to demographic and academic attributes (e.g., place of birth, age, last school grade in German language) which are considered to be important for social integration (similarity attraction hypothesis)?
- Do children from various immigrant groups differ from each other and from native borns in direct and indirect forms of bullying?
- Are there differences in friendship patterns and peer acceptance between native children and immigrant children from various countries of origin?

METHOD

Procedure and Participants

Research was conducted in 29 classes (6th and 7th grades) of six general secondary schools situated in a middle-sized city in the southern part of Austria.[1] General secondary schools serve predominantly lower-middle-class families, and show higher aggression levels of pupils than academic secondary schools (e.g., Gasteiger-Klicpera & Klicpera, 1997). In the present study general secondary schools with a considerably high amount of immigrant children were investigated.

Participation in the study was voluntary; strict confidentiality for both pupils and schools was guaranteed. After the study was accepted by the local school council, school principals provided alphabetic class rosters of participating classes. Based on these rosters, every child was assigned to a code. These rosters were projected onto the wall in the classrooms during data collection. While filling in the questionnaire pupils were asked to use the presented codes instead of names to assure their confidentiality. Data collection was done by two trained bilingual (German and Serbian/Croatian and Turkish) research assistants during a regular lesson and lasted about 2 hours.

In sum, 326 native and 242 immigrant children (258 girls and 310 boys) participated in the study. According to the official statistics of the local school council, 886 pupils of general secondary schools in this district were immigrant children (Kerschbaumer, 2000). That means, 27% of the population of immigrant children who attended a general secondary school in this school district participated in the study. The children of the immigrant subsample spoke 22 different mother-tongues which were shown to represent the population well. For theoretical and practical reasons participants were divided into four groups: native children (57%), children from the former Yugoslavia (22%), Turkish and Kurdish children (14%), and a heterogeneous rest group (7%). Whereas children of the first three groups are considered as similar regarding their cultural backgrounds, children of the rest group are mostly the only representatives of their immigrant group in the schoolclass and thus are considered as similar with respect to their social situation. We acknowledge that the group labels are imprecise and that there is additional heterogeneity within these categories. However, it is likely that these broad categories, rather than more narrow subgroups, are particularly salient to the peer group. Similar group distinctions were made by Hanish and Guerra (2000a, 2000b) for various ethnic groups in the U.S.

INSTRUMENTS

Bully/Victim Behavior

In the present study "bullying" was defined according to Olweus (1993). Because of the fact that an exact translation of the term "bullying" into German is not possible (Spiel & Atria, 2001; Spiel, 2000; Strohmeier & Spiel, 2000) instead of an ambiguous translation the English term "bullying" was used and was explained to the pupils in a very careful and standardized way. In addition, participants were presented with the German version of the definition of "bullying" provided in the Olweus Bullying Inventory (1989).[2]

Self-ratings. Participants were presented with four subscales of the Bully/ Victim Questionnaire (BVQ; Olweus, 1989). Previously checks of psycho- metric properties of the German version of these subscales showed satisfying results. Reliability estimates (Cronbach's alphas) ranged between .61 and .85 (Robier, 1997; Singer, 1998). The subscales are: (1) Victim Scale of Indirect Bullying (4 items; example: How much do you like recess time?), (2) Victim Scale of Direct Bullying (4 items; example: How often have you been bullied at school this term?), (3) Bully Scale (5 items; example: How often have you taken part in bullying other young people at school this term?), and (4) Attitude to Bullying Scale (3 items; example: What do you think about pupils who join in bullying other young people?). The response scales in this inventory are paraphrased verbally and range from 1 (low feature characteristic) to 5 (high feature characteristic). Several of the response alternatives are fairly specific, such as "about once a week," and "several times a week" and thus, more objec- tive than alternatives like "often" and "very often."

Peer ratings. According to the definition of "bullying" provided in the BVQ (Olweus, 1989; see above) participants were asked to nominate every classmate they regarded (1) as a bully and/or (2) as a victim. To control for the varying class-sizes (ranged between 16 and 27 pupils) participants were classi- fied as "victims" or "bullies," when they were nominated by more than 33% of their classmates. Similar cut-off points were used, e.g., by Boulton and Smith (1994) and Salmivalli, Huttunen, and Lagerspetz (1997).

Friendship Patterns and Peer Acceptance

To assess children's level of peer acceptance a sociometric nomination technique was used (Coie, Dodge, & Copotelli, 1982). Self-ratings were ap- plied to get insights into participants' friendship patterns.

Self-ratings. Participants were asked to write down name, country of origin, and gender of their friends (both classmates and others). They were requested to think of a person as a "friend" if they like that person very much, feel emo- tionally close to that person, spend lots of their leisure time with that person, tell secrets to that person and if they think that their lives would be very differ- ent without that person. For each child, the number of friends differentiated by her/his country of origin (Austria, former Yugoslavia, Turkey and other coun- tries) was calculated.

Peer ratings. Participants were asked to nominate the three classmates they liked most (LM) and the three classmates they liked least (LL). Based on this information these two indicators were combined to a "social preference (SP)" score (SP = LM-LL; see Peery, 1979). Social preference scores are used to in- dex a child's actual peer acceptance (number of positive nominations minus number of negative nominations). Sociometric classifications based on social preference scores were shown to exhibit good one-year stability (Coie & Dodge, 1983). To control for the varying class sizes, the measure was z-standardized by class.

In addition, information about demographic and academic attributes considered to be important for the social integration of immigrant children was collected (Berscheid, 1985; Laireiter & Baumann, 1992). These variables are: age, place of birth, mid-term marks in German language, mother-tongue instruction, and duration of stay in Austria.[3]

RESULTS

In the first step, children from the three immigrant groups were compared in demographic and academic attributes. Results of analyses are shown in Table 1.

Univariate ANOVAS, χ^2 tests, and Alpha corrected Bonferroni post hoc tests showed that age, place of birth, mid-term marks in German language, duration of stay in Austria and the attendance of additional mother-tongue instruction are not equal between groups (see Table 1). Turkish and Kurdish children were older than children of the other groups, $F_{(3/559)} = 11.54$, $p < 0.001$. Furthermore, Turkish and Kurdish children and children of the rest group achieved lower marks in German compared to Austrians and children from the former Yugoslavia, $F_{(3/539)} =$

TABLE 1. Description of Immigrant and Native Children

Groups of children	Native children		Rest group children		Turkish/Kurdish children		Children of the former Yugoslavia	
Age	M	SD	M	SD	M	SD	M	SD
	12.70	0.97	12.89	1.06	13.42	0.93	12.71	1.05
Place of birth	AUSTRIA	elsewhere	AUSTRIA	elsewhere	AUSTRIA	elsewhere	AUSTRIA	elsewhere
	n = 324	n = 2	n = 6	n = 30	n = 1	n = 79	n = 16	n = 110
	99.4%	0.6%	16.7%	83.3%	1.2%	98.8%	12.7%	87.3%
Mid-term marks in German language	M	SD	M	SD	M	SD	M	SD
	3.12	0.94	3.83	1.41	3.92	1.25	3.19	0.92
Mother-tongue instruction			yes	no	yes	no	yes	no
			n = 12	n = 23	n = 41	n = 38	n = 19	n = 105
			34.3%	65.7%	51.9%	48.1%	15.3%	84.7%
Duration of stay in Austria (in months)			M	SD	M	SD	M	SD
			69.67	55.45	52.29	34.07	94.11	34.63

16.59, p < 0.001. Children of the former Yugoslavia and children of the rest group were more often born in Austria than Turkish children, χ^2 (2) = 9.98, p < 0.01. In addition, children of the former Yugoslavia stayed longer in Austria than Turkish children and children of the rest group, F (2/235) = 29.49, p < 0.001. In addition, groups differed with respect to additional mother-tongue instruction: 52% of the Turkish children, 34% of the rest group children and 15% of the children from the former Yugoslavia attended these voluntary lessons, χ^2 (2) = 30.91, p < 0.001.

PROBLEMATIC INTERETHNIC INTERACTIONS

Bully/Victim Status: Peer-Ratings

In sum, 9.1% of the participants were classified as bullies and 6.7% as victims. Statistically significant differences between immigrant and native born children were found in the distribution of both bullies, χ^2 (3) = 7.77, p = 0.05, and victims, χ^2 (3) = 8.13, p = 0.04. Thus, 11.8% of the native Austrian, 7.2% of the former Yugoslavian, but only 3.8% of the Turkish/Kurdish and 2.8% of the rest group children were classified as bullies. For the victim status a slightly different picture emerged: 9.0% of the native Austrian, 8.3% of the rest group, 5.1% of the Turkish/Kurdish and only 1.6% of the former Yugoslavian children were identified as victims based on peer-ratings.

Bully/Victim Behavior: Self-Ratings

To make reliable comparisons between the groups of children, the psychometric properties of the Bully/Victim Questionnaire (Olweus, 1989) in native and all groups of immigrant children were checked.

For each group, the internal consistency of the four subscales of the BVQ was examined using Cronbach's alphas. Analyses revealed satisfying consistency scores for all groups of children in the Victim Scale of Direct Bullying, the Bully Scale and the Attitude to Bullying Scale (Cronbach's ranged between 0.54 and 0.83). However, striking differences in internal consistency were found for the Victim Scale of Indirect Bullying between native children and all groups of immigrant children (see Table 2).

As shown in Table 2, item total correlations were very low in the subsamples of immigrant children. Thus, the concept of indirect aggression, defined as (1) liking recess times; (2) feeling lonely at school; (3) being alone during recess times; and (4) being as well liked as the other students in class (Olweus, 1989) does not fit to immigrant children.

TABLE 2. Olweus Scale of Indirect Bullying–Internal Consistencies (α) and Item Reliabilities (*rit*) for Groups of Children

Reliability scores	Groups of children			
	Native children	Rest group children	Turkish / Kurdish children	Children of the former Yugoslavia
How do you like recess time?	.20	−.01	−.09	.05
Do you feel lonely at school?	.55	.25	.04	.44
How often does it happen that other students don't want to spend recess time with you and you end up being alone?	.46	.40	.15	.39
Do you feel you are less well liked than other students in your class?	.44	.16	−.01	.15
Internal consistency (Cronbach Alpha's of Scale)	.63	.36	.04	.44

When investigating differences in bully/victim behavior between immigrant and native children, results of psychometric analyses were taken into account. First, we conducted a 2 × 4 MANOVA with gender and group (native Austrian, former Yugoslavian, Turkish/Kurdish, and rest group) as factors and the three internally consistent subscale scores of the BVQ (Victim Scale of Direct Bullying, Bully Scale and Attitude to Bullying Scale) as dependent variables. Application of multivariate tests using Pilais Criterion did neither identify a main effect group nor an interaction effect. However, a gender effect was observed, $F(3,539) = 3.59$, $p = 0.02$, $\eta^2 = 0.02$. Follow-up univariate tests revealed differences between boys and girls regarding the Attitude to Bullying Scale, $F(1,541) = 7.20$, $p < 0.01$, $\eta^2 = 0.01$. Boys reported more positive attitudes towards bullying (M = 7.49, SD = 3.06) than girls did (M = 6.77, SD = 2.77).

To explore differences in indirect forms of bullying a second 2 × 4 MANOVA with the factors gender and group and the four single items of the Victim Scale of Indirect Bullying as dependent variables was conducted. Multivariate tests using Pilais Criterion identified both main effects group, $F(12,1647) = 5.91$, $p < 0.001$, $\eta^2 = 0.04$, and gender, $F(4,547) = 4.59$, $p < 0.001$, $\eta^2 = 0.03$, to be significant. No significant interaction was found. Follow-up univariate tests revealed differences between immigrant groups in the items "How do you like recess times?," $F(3,550) = 3.32$, $p = 0.02$, $\eta^2 = 0.02$, and "Do you feel lonely at school?," $F(3,550) = 11.52$, $p < 0.001$, $\eta^2 = 0.06$. Alpha corrected Bonferroni post hoc tests showed that Turkish/Kurdish children liked recess less (M = 1.54, SD = 1.08) than native children (M = 1.23, SD = 0.69). Furthermore, Turkish/Kurdish children (M = 2.35, SD = 1.38), and rest group children (M = 2.17, SD = 1.07) reported to feel more often lonely at school than native (M = 1.68, SD = 0.86) and former Yugoslavian children (M = 1.69, SD = 1.02).

COOPERATIVE FORMS OF INTERETHNIC INTERACTIONS

Peer Acceptance

To compare the four groups (native Austrian, former Yugoslavian, Turkish/Kurdish, and rest group) in peer acceptance a 2 × 4 ANOVA was conducted with the standardized social acceptance score as dependent variable and gender and group as factors. The two main effects, gender, $F(1,554) = 4.73$, p = 0.03, $\eta^2 = 0.01$, and group, $F(3,554) = 5.70$, p = 0.02, $\eta^2 = 0.03$, were shown to be statistically significant. Alpha corrected Bonferroni post hoc tests revealed that Turkish/Kurdish children (M = −0.46, SD = 0.96) were less accepted by their peers than both native (M = 0.06, SD = 1.00) and former Yugoslavian children (M = 0.14, SD = 0.84). Furthermore, boys (M = −0.10, SD = 1.04) were less accepted than girls (M = 0.12, SD = 0.87).

Friendship Patterns

On average, 68.52% of the friends nominated by the participants were their classmates. In this percentage no group differences were found. To compare the four groups (native Austrian, former Yugoslavian, Turkish/Kurdish, and rest group) in their nomination of classmates as friends a 2 × 4 ANOVA was conducted with gender and group as factors and the number of classmates nominated as friends as dependent variable. The main effect group, $F(3,547) = 5.97$, p < 0.001, $\eta^2 = 0.03$, appeared to be statistically significant. Post hoc tests according to Bonferroni revealed that Turkish/Kurdish children nominated fewer classmates as friends (M = 2.71, SD = 2.47) than did native (M = 4.00, SD = 2.87) and former Yugoslavian children (M = 4.50, SD = 3.29).

To get insights in children's interethnic friendship patterns, the total number of Austrian, former Yugoslavian, Turkish/Kurdish, and other friends were counted for each participant. A repeated measures MANOVA with the country of origin of the friends (Austria, former Yugoslavia, Turkey, other countries) as the within subject factor and the own group membership (native, former Yugoslavia, Turkish/Kurdish, and rest group) as the between subject factor was conducted. The number of friends was used as dependent variable. Multivariate tests using Pilais Criterion showed a significant main effect on the within factor country of origin of friends, $F(3,562) = 84.24$, p < 0.001, $\eta^2 =$

0.31, and a significant interaction effect, $F(9,1692) = 56.78$, $p < 0.001$, $\eta^2 = 0.23$. The between factor group was also statistically significant, $F(3,564) = 17.08$, $p = 0.01$, $\eta^2 = 0.02$.

As shown in Figure 1, children had specific friendship patterns depending on their group membership. Whereas native and Turkish/Kurdish children showed a strong preference for friends from their own group, this was not the case for children of the former Yugoslavia and of the rest group.

DISCUSSION

The focus of the present study lay on the investigation of both negative and positive aspects of interethnic interactions of children from various countries of origin in ethnically mixed school classes. In particular, we compared prevalence rates of bullying (for both victims and perpetrators) in native and immigrant children, which were divided into three groups (former Yugoslavia, Turkish/Kurdish, heterogeneous rest group). We also investigated direct and indirect forms of bullying, peer acceptance and friendship patterns in native borns and children of the three immigrant groups. Results provide support for the hypothesis that interethnic interactions of children vary systematically depending on their country of origin.

FIGURE 1. Interethnic Friendship Patterns

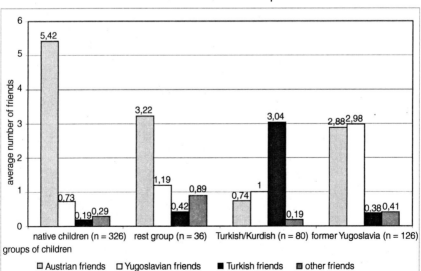

Prevalence Rates of Bullying

The design of the present study differs in several aspects from previous studies on peer aggression in immigrant children (e.g., Loesel et al., 1999; Popp, 2000; Klicpera & Gasteiger-Klicpera, 1996; Fuchs, 1999). *First*, immigrant children were not uniformly labeled as one homogeneous group of "foreign children," but were distinguished into three immigrant groups. Contrary to the majority of previous studies, primary analyses were conducted to check for particularities regarding demographic and academic attributes between groups. Data suggest that children of various immigrant groups differ considerably from each other. Analyses revealed that children of the former Yugoslavia are more similar to natives than other immigrants. *Second*, bullying according to Olweus (1993) was examined not only via self-ratings but also via nomination techniques. Peer ratings are considered as reliable and valid data source and nomination techniques are frequently used (e.g., Schuster, 1999; Salmivalli et al., 1996; Perry, Kusel, & Perry, 1988). *Third*, to reliably identify victims and perpetrators of bullying and to control for varying class-sizes rather a strict criterion was used. A child was labeled as "bully" and/or "victim" if he/she was identified by more than 33% of his/her classmates.

In sum, 9% of the children were found to be bullies and 7% to be victims. Analyses revealed that native children were more often nominated as victims (9%) and perpetrators (12%) than all subgroups of immigrant children. This result indicates that bullying is rather a problem of the native than of the immigrant children. These findings support results of a study conducted in the U.S. Hanish and Guerra (2000b) showed that children of the host society (European-American and African-American) were at higher risk for peer victimization than Hispanic immigrant children.

Measuring Indirect Bullying in Immigrant Children

In the present study, indirect bullying was defined under the terms of social exclusion (Olweus, 1989) and measured via self-ratings. Analyses of the psychometric properties of the Victim Scale of Indirect Bullying showed insufficient reliability estimates for all subsamples of immigrant children. Additional analyses revealed that the items of the scale do not build a homogeneous construct in immigrant children. Thus, we recommend not to investigate indirect aggression in immigrant children with scales which compound questions about feelings of loneliness and problematic social relationships. It seems to be more fruitful to ask for social risk factors in immigrant children as defined by Hodges, Malone, and Perry (1997), that is, lacking supportive friends and being rejected by the peer group.

Social Risk Factors in Immigrant Children

To measure social risk factors in the present study, we investigated social acceptance, number of friends, and cross-cultural friendship patterns (e.g., Hodges, Malone, & Perry, 1997). Only Turkish/Kurdish children were shown to be at risk concerning their social relationships. They were low accepted by their peers, felt most lonely at school and had fewer friends in class than native children and children from other immigrant groups. In the literature, the main causes for peer rejection (and low acceptance) are seen either in a higher aggression level (e.g., Parker & Asher, 1987) or in a social skill deficit (e.g., Putallaz & Gottmann, 1981) of the rejected child. Findings of Rost and Czeschlik (1994) and Vedder and O'Dowd (1999) emphasized the importance of verbal comprehension for peer acceptance. Because of the fact that Turkish and Kurdish immigrant children were less likely to be nominated as bullies in the present study, we suggest that lack of "cultural skills" (e.g., lack of language proficiency, different behavior because of different cultural norms) could be an important factor which may contribute to higher social risk in immigrant children. This hypothesis might be supported by the observation that Yugoslavian children which were shown to be more similar to Austrians than the other immigrant children had no problems with respect to their social relationships. Moreover, they established cross-cultural friendships more frequently than both native children and children from the other immigrant groups.

To prove this hypothesis and to explain the observed differences in interethnic interactions, further research is needed. As we found remarkable differences in peer acceptance and friendship patterns in children depending on their country of origin, we recommend distinguishing immigrant children in even more than three groups. As a consequence, however, large samples have to be collected.

Findings of the present study suggest that social risk factors are not equally distributed in the four groups of children. Whereas native Austrians are more likely to be engaged in direct forms of bullying, Turkish/Kurdish children seem to have a lack in cooperative forms of interactions. These findings have to be taken into account when applying interventions in multicultural school classes. In any case, training of social skills, sensitization for differences in behavior of children depending on their country of origin, as well as activities promoting a common identity are recommended.

As the present study is limited because of its cross-sectional design, longitudinal studies are recommended to get insights in the development of interethnic interactions in multicultural school classes. In future research, demographic and academic characteristics of immigrant children (e.g., duration of stay, language proficiency) as well as structural variables of the social environment (e.g., the ratio of immigrant children in the classrooms), should be investigated systematically.

NOTES

1. In Austria, compulsory schooling starts with a child's sixth birthday and lasts nine school years. In the first four years the attendance of a primary school is obligatory. After the primary school children can attend either a general secondary school (5th to 8th grade) or an academic secondary school (5th to 12th grade).

2. "Here are some questions about bullying. We say a student is being bullied when another student, or a group of students, say nasty and unpleasant things to him or her. It is also bullying when a student is hit, kicked, threatened, locked inside a room, and things like that. These things may take place frequently and it is difficult for the student being bullied to defend himself or herself. It is also bullying when a student is teased repeatedly in a negative way. But it is not bullying when two students of about the same strength quarrel or fight" (p. 2).

3. In Austria, school marks range from 1 (excellent) to 5 (failed). Mother-tongue instruction is an additional voluntary lesson for immigrant children to learn their first language.

REFERENCES

Berry, J. W. (1980). Acculturation as varieties of adaptation. In A. Padilla (Ed.), *Acculturation, theory, models and some new findings*. Boulder, CO: Westview Press.

Berscheid, E. (1985). Interpersonal attraction. In G. Lindzey & E. Aronson (Eds.), *Handbook of social psychology* (pp. 413-484). New York: Random House.

Bjoerqvist, K., Lagerspetz, K. M. J., & Kaukiainen, A. (1992). Do girls manipulate and boys fight? Developmental trends in regard to direct and indirect aggression. *Aggressive Behavior*, 18, 117-127.

Boulton, M. J. & Smith, P. K. (1996). Liking and peer perceptions among Asian and white British children. *Journal of Social and Personal Relationships*, 13, 163-177.

Boulton, M. J. & Smith, P. K. (1994). Bully/victim problems in middle-school children: Stability, self-perceived competence, peer-perceptions and peer acceptance. *British Journal of Developmental Psychology*, 12, 315-329.

Bourhis, R. Y., Moise, C. L., Perreault, S. & Senecal, S. (1997). Towards an interactive acculturation model: A social psychological approach. *International Journal of Psychology*, 32 (6), 369-386.

Brown, B. B. (1990). Peer groups and peer cultures. In S. Feldman & G. Elliott (Eds.), *At the threshold* (pp. 171-196). Cambridge, MA: Havard University Press.

Brown, R. (1995). *Prejudice. Its Social Psychology*. Oxford: Blackwell.

Bukowski, W. M. & Hoza, B. (1989). Popularity and friendship: Issues in theory, measurement and outcomes. In T. Berndt & G. Ladd (Eds.), *Peer relations in child development*. New York, Wiley.

Coie, J. D. & Dodge, K. A. (1983). Continuities and changes in children's sociometric status: A five-year longitudinal study. *Merrill-Palmer Quarterly*, 29, 261-282.

Coie, J. D., Dodge, K. A., & Coppotelli, H. (1982). Dimensions and types of social status: A cross age perspective. *Developmental Psychology*, 18(4), 557-570.

Crick, N. & Grotpeter, J. K. (1995). Relational aggression, gender, and social-psychological adjustment. *Child Development*, 66, 710-722.

Fuchs, M. (1999). Ausländische Schüler und Gewalt an Schulen. Ergebnisse einer Schüler- und Lehrerbefragung. [Foreign pupils and violence at school: Results of a pupil and teacher survey.] In Holtappels, H. G., Heitmeyer W., Melzer, W., & Tillmann, K. (Hrsg.) *Forschung über Gewalt an Schulen. Erscheinungsformen, Ursachen, Konzepte und Prävention. [Research about violence in schools: Manifestations, causes, concepts and prevention.]* (S. 119-136). Weinheim, München: Juventa Verlag.

Gasteiger-Klicpera, B. & Klicpera, C. (1997). Aggressivität und soziale Stellung in der Klassengemeinschaft. [Aggressiveness and social status in the classroom.] *Zeitschrift für Kinder- und Jugendpsychiatrie*, 25, 139-150.

Graham, J. A. & Cohen, R. (1997). Race and gender as factors in children's sociometric ratings and friendship choices. *Social Development*, 6(3), 355-372.

Graham, J. A., Cohen, R., Zbikowski, S. M., & Secrist, M. E. (1998). A longitudinal investigation of race and gender as factors in children's classroom friendship choices. *Child Study Journal*, 28(4), 245-266.

Hanish, L. D. & Guerra, N. G. (2000a). Predictors of peer victimization among urban youth. *Social Development*, 9(4), 521-543.

Hanish, L. D. & Guerra, N. G. (2000b). The roles of ethnicity and school context in predicting children's victimization by peers. *American Journal of Community Psychology*, 28 (2), 201-223.

Hodges, E., Malone, M. & Perry, D. (1997). Individual risk and social risk as interacting determinants of victimization in the peer group. *Developmental Psychology*, 33 (6), 1032-1039.

Kerschbaumer, G. (2000). *Schüler/innen nichtdeutscher Muttersprache an den allgemein bildenden Pflichtschulen der steirischen Schulbezirke. Daten zum Stichtag 30.9.1999. Offizielle Statistik des Grazer Stadtschulamtes, Schulberatungsstelle für Ausländer. [Pupils with non-German mother-tongues in public schools in Styria. Due date: September, 30, 1999.* Official statistics of the School Council of Graz, Information Center for Foreigners.]

Klicpera, C. & Gasteiger-Klicpera, B. (1996). Die Situation von "Tätern" und "Opfern" aggressiver Handlungen in der Schule. [The situation of "perpetrators" and "victims" of aggressive acts at school.] *Praxis Kinderpsychologie und Kinderpsychiatrie*, 45 (1), 2-9.

Kupersmidt, J. B., DeRosier, M. E., & Patterson, C. P. (1995). Similarity as the basis for children's friendships: The roles of sociometric status, aggressive and withdrawn behavior, academic achievement, and demographic characteristics. *Journal of Social and Personal Relationships*, 12, 439-452.

Lagerspetz, K. M. J., Bjoerqvist, J., & Peltonen, T. (1988). Is indirect aggression typical of females? Gender differences in aggressiveness in 11- to 12-year-old children. *Aggressive Behavior*, 14, 403-414.

Lagerspetz, K. M. J., & Bjoerqvist, K. (1994). Indirect aggression in boys and girls. In L. R. Huesmann (Ed.), *Aggressive behavior: Current perspectives* (pp. 131-150). New York: Plenum.

Laireiter, A. & Baumann, U. (1992). Network structures and support functions: Theoretical and empirical analyses. In H.O.F. Veil & U. Baumann (Eds.), *The meaning and measurement of social support* (pp. 33-55). Washington: Hemisphere.

Loesel, F., Bliesener T., & Averbeck, M. (1999). Hat die Delinquenz von Schülern zugenommen? Ein Vergleich im Dunkelfeld. [Has delinquency risen in pupils?] In Schäfer, M. & Frey, D. (Hrsg.) *Aggression und Gewalt unter Kindern und Jugendlichen. [Aggression and violence in children and adolescents.]* (S. 65-90) Göttingen, Bern, Toronto, Seattle: Hogrefe, Verlag für Psychologie.

Maccoby, E. E. (1988). Gender as a social category. *Developmental Psychology*, 24, 755-765.

Maccoby, E. E. (1990). Gender and relationships: A developmental account. *American Psychologist*, 45, 513-520.

Maharaj, S. I. & Connolly, J. A. (1994). Peer network composition of acculturated and ethnoculturally affiliated adolescents in a multicultural setting. *Journal of Adolescent Research*, 9 (2), 218-240.

Olweus, D. (1989). *The Olweus Bully/Victim Questionnaire*. Mimeograph. Bergen, Norway.

Olweus, D. (1993). *Bullying at School: What We Know and What We Can Do*. Oxford: Blackwell.

Parker, J. G. & Asher, S. R. (1987). Peer relations and later personal adjustment. Are low-accepted children at risk? *Psychological Bulletin*, 102 (3), 357-389.

Peery, J. C. (1979). Popular, amiable, isolated, rejected: A reconceptualization of sociometric status in preschool children. *Child Development*, 50, 1231-1234.

Perry, D. G., Kusel, S. J., & Perry, L. C. (1988). Victims of peer aggression. *Developmental Psychology*, 24, 807-814.

Popp, U. (2000). Gewalt an Schulen als "Türkenproblem?" Gewaltniveau, Wahrnehmung von Klassenklima und sozialer Diskriminierung bei deutschen und türkischen Schülerinnen und Schülern. [Violence in schools as a problem of the Turkish pupils? Acts of violence, perception of the social climate in learning groups and social discrimination by German and Turkish pupils.] *Empirische Pädagogik*, 14 (1), 59-91.

Putallaz, M. & Gottman, J. M. (1981). Social skills and group acceptance. In S. R. Asher & J. M. Gottman (Eds.), *The development of children's friendships* (pp. 116-149). New York: Cambridge University Press.

Robier, C. (1997). *Aggressionsbekämpfung in Hauptschulen. Zum Einfluss von Angst und Gewalt im Fernsehen. [Tackling aggression in general secondary schools: On the influence of anxiety and violence at TV.]* Unpublished master thesis, University of Graz, Austria.

Rost, D. H. & Czeschlik, T. (1994). Beliebt und intelligent? Abgelehnt und dumm? Eine soziometrische Studie an 6,500 Grundschulkindern [Popular and intelligent? Rejected and dumb? A sociometric study with 6,500 primary school pupils]. *Zeitschrift für Sozialpsychologie*, 1994, S. 170-176.

Rys, G. S. & Bear, G. G. (1997). Relational aggression and peer relations: Gender and developmental issues. *Merrill-Palmer Quarterly*, 43(1), 87-106.

Salmivalli, C., Huttunen, A., & Lagerspetz, K. M. J. (1997). Peer networks and bullying in schools. *Scandinavian Journal of Psychology*, 38, 305-312.

Salmivalli, C., Lagerspetz, K., Bjoerkqvist, K. & Oestermann, K., (1996). Bullying as a group process: Participant roles and their relations to social status within the group. *Aggressive Behavior*, 22 (1), 1-15.

Schuster, B. (1999). Outsiders at school: The prevalence of bullying and its relation with social status. *Group Processes and Intergroup Relations*, Vol. 2 (2), 175-190.

Singer, M. (1998). *Anwendung des Anti-Aggressionsprogramms nach Dan Olweus an österreichischen Schulen. Zusammenhänge zwischen Aggression, Klassen- und Familienklima.* [*Implementation of the anti-bullying program according to Dan Olweus at Austrian schools. Correlations between aggression, class- and family climate.*] Unpublished master thesis, University of Graz, Austria.

Spiel, C. (2000). Gewalt in der Schule: Täter, Opfer, Prävention-Intervention. In Tatzer, E., Pflanzer, S., & Krisch, K. (Eds.), *Schlimm verletzt. Schwierige Kinder und Jugendliche in Theorie und Praxis* (pp. 41-53). Wien: Krammer. [Violence at school: Bullies, victims, prevention-intervention. In Tatzer, E., Pflanzer, S. & Krisch, K. (Eds.), *Badly injured. Difficult children and adolescents in theory and praxis.*]

Spiel, C. & Atria, M. (2001). *Tackling Violence in Schools: A Report from Austria.* Retrieved March, 30, 2002, from http://www.goldsmiths.ac.uk/connect/reportaustria.html

Strohmeier, D. & Spiel, C. (2000, 17.-18.11.2000). *Gewalterfahrungen von Kindern unterschiedlicher Muttersprachen–Eine Studie an Grazer Hauptschulen.* [*Violence experiences of children with various mother-tongues–Preliminary results of a study conducted in general secondary schools in Graz.*]. Paper presented at the 5th workshop on "aggression" in Hannover, Germany.

Strohmeier, D. & Spiel, C. (2001, 9.-10.11.2001). *Aussenseiter in der Schule. Bullying als Gruppenphänomen.* [*Outsiders at school. Bullying as a group phenomenon.*]. Paper presented at the 6th workshop on "aggression" in Jena, Germany.

Sutton, J. & Smith, P. K. (1999). Bullying as a group process: An adaptation of the participant role approach. *Aggressive Behavior*, 25 (2), 97-111.

Vedder, P. & O'Dowd (1999). Swedish primary school pupils' inter-ethnic relationships. *Scandinavian Journal of Psychology*, 40, 221-228.

Peer Victimization in Middle School: When Self- and Peer Views Diverge

Sandra Graham
Amy Bellmore
Jaana Juvonen

University of California, Los Angeles

SUMMARY. African American ($n = 350$) and Latino ($n = 435$) 6th grade students from eight middle schools completed self-report measures of peer victimization and psychological adjustment (i.e., self-esteem, anxiety, loneliness, depression, and physical symptoms). Peer nomination procedures were used to determine which students had reputations as victims and which students were accepted, rejected, and perceived as most "cool." In addition, homeroom teachers rated participating students on social behavior and academic engagement and students' grades were collected from school records. We created four victim groups based on self- and peer perceptions. "True" victims (agreement between self and peer) experienced the worst outcomes on all of the adjustment variables examined. However, different adjustment difficulties were reported for victim groups where there was disagreement between self- and peer views. Self-perceived victimization was predictive of psychological maladjustment, whereas the reputational measure was

---

Address correspondence to: Sandra Graham, Department of Education, University of California, Los Angeles, CA 90095-1521 (E-mail: shgraham@ucla.edu).

[Haworth co-indexing entry note]: "Peer Victimization in Middle School: When Self- and Peer Views Diverge." Graham, Sandra, Amy Bellmore, and Jaana Juvonen. Co-published simultaneously in *Journal of Applied School Psychology* (The Haworth Press, Inc.) Vol. 19, No. 2, 2003, pp. 117-137; and: *Bullying, Peer Harassment, and Victimization in the Schools: The Next Generation of Prevention* (ed: Maurice J. Elias, and Joseph E. Zins) The Haworth Press, Inc., 2003, pp. 117-137. Single or multiple copies of this article are available for a fee from The Haworth Document Delivery Service [1-800-HAWORTH, 9:00 a.m. - 5:00 p.m. (EST). E-mail address: docdelivery@ haworthpress.com].

10.1300/J008v19n02_08

more related to peer rejection and negative teacher ratings. The implications of the findings for both accurate identification of victims of harassment and targeted intervention strategies were discussed. *[Article copies available for a fee from the Haworth Document Delivery Service: 1-800-HAWORTH. E-mail address: <docdelivery@haworthpress.com> Website: <http://www. HaworthPress.com> © 2003 by the Haworth Press, Inc. All rights reserved.]*

KEYWORDS. Identification, ethnic differences, adjustment, intervention

A common theme underlying the articles on peer victimization in this volume is the vulnerability of those children and adolescents who are chronically picked on by others. Even more than their perpetrators, the targets of peer hostility face numerous mental health challenges and they are particularly at risk for social and emotional adjustment problems (see Nansel et al., 2001 for a recent review). Unfortunately, many cases of peer harassment go undetected because students are unwilling to talk about getting picked on at school. As a result, school professionals sometimes find themselves dealing with the symptoms of chronic harassment (e.g., feelings of anxiety and depression) before they learn about their cause. An important task for psychologists and other adults in the school setting is, therefore, to accurately identify those students whose adjustment difficulties are due to victimization by peers.

How do school personnel know which students are victims of peer harassment? Experience might suggest a simple answer to that question. Just ask the students. Survey their peers. Or simply observe for yourself. Yet accurate identification of children who are victims of peer harassment is more complex than simply asking, surveying, or observing. That is because each informant source produces a particular kind of data that has its own limitations. Self-reports of victimization are subjective experiences that are privately felt and are not necessarily verifiable by other informants. One particularly painful experience may have far reaching effects on self-perceived victim status, just as multiple experiences with harassment may be discounted as a strategy to protect one's self-esteem. In other words, subjective disclosures of feeling like a victim are prone to all of the biases (e.g., underestimating, overestimating) that are associated with self-report data. Peer data produce reputational measures of victimization; they reflect agreement or consensus among peers about the relative standing of individuals compared to other members of the group. Because social reputations, once entrenched, are highly resistant to change, using peers as informants is subject to any of the biases or judgment errors that are associated with making inferences about others (Hymel, Wagner, & Butler,

1990). Observational data may be the least reliable source of information because much of peer harassment is covert. At least by middle school, the most common forms of harassment typically occur in "unowned" (and unseen) school spaces, such as bathrooms, hallways, and locker rooms where adult supervision is minimal (Astor, Meyer, & Behre, 1999).

In light of these reliability concerns, it is surprising that the issue of informant source has not received much attention in the peer harassment literature (but see Pelligrini, 2001 for a notable exception). Most studies have used either self-reports (e.g., "Are *you* someone who gets picked on by others?") or peer nominations (e.g., "Which kids in your class get picked on by others?"). Typically self-reports yield higher estimates of peer harassment than do peer reports (Schuster, 1996). Studies that use only one method may, therefore, be under- or over-identifying students who are truly victimized (Juvonen, Nishina, & Graham, 2001). Or they may overlook important differences between victimized youth for whom self- and peer views diverge. For example, might there be different concerns for victims who view themselves as harassed but have no such reputation among peers, compared to those who carry a reputation that they themselves do not endorse?

We documented some of those differences in a recent study that examined self-report and peer nomination victim data in a sample of middle-school students (Graham & Juvonen, 1998). We identified four victim groups that took into account self- and peer views. Two groups enjoyed complete agreement between self and peers: those were nonvictims (low victim scores from both informants) and "true" victims (high scores from both). A third group was high on self-perceived victimization, but did not have that reputation based on peer reports. We labeled that group self-identified victims. A fourth group, labeled peer-identified victims, did not perceive themselves as victims but had that reputation among their peers.

When comparing the victim groups across psychological and social adjustment indices, we found that particular patterns of adjustment were systematically related to different types of victims. Self-identified victims reported as much loneliness, anxiety, and low self-esteem as did true victims, but they were not more rejected by peers than nonvictims. Peer-identified victims, on the other hand, were just as rejected as true victims, but their self-views were no more negative than those of nonvictims. Those findings suggested that self-views about victimization might be more predictive of psychological maladjustment, whereas peer views might be more predictive of social maladjustment. That distinction is important because most victimization studies describe a cluster of adjustment difficulties–including loneliness, anxiety, *and* peer rejection–without considering whether particular problems are more linked to particular types of identification methods.

In the research reported here, we further explored differences between victim subgroups based on self- and peer reports with a larger middle-school sample and an expanded set of adjustment outcomes, including depression and physical symptoms. We also gathered data on teacher ratings of student academic and social behavior to determine whether the appraisals of third party informants conform more closely to self-views or peer views. In addition, data on academic performance of students were collected from school records. A number of studies have reported a relationship between peer victimization and school problems (e.g., Juvonen, Nishina, & Graham, 2000; Kochenderfer & Ladd, 1996). However, it is unclear whether the peer harassment-low achievement linkage is the same or different for students who subjectively experience victimization versus those who only have that reputation among their peers. Examining different types of victims and their unique adjustment difficulties can provide useful information for professional staff as well as researchers working in school settings. That information relates to both identification (i.e., how do adults in the school know when someone is a victim of harassment?) and intervention (i.e., should school personnel be tailoring specific types of intervention strategies to specific victim types?).

METHOD

Participants

Participants were 785 sixth-grade students (348 boys and 437 girls, M age = 11.5 yrs) recruited from eight middle schools in metropolitan Los Angeles. The sample for this study was selected from a larger cohort of sixth graders (n = 1,223; 45% Latino, 39% African-American, 6% Caucasian, 5% Asian, 5% from other ethnic groups) who were taking part in a longitudinal investigation of peer relations during the middle-school years. To examine the possibility of ethnic group differences in victim subtypes, we included participants from only the two largest ethnic groups; that is, Latinos (n = 435; 205 boys, 230 girls) and African Americans (n = 350; 143 boys, 207 girls). In terms of immigrant history, 90% of the Latino youth were at least second generation (U.S. born children of immigrants) and all were sufficiently proficient in English to complete the surveys. The eight participating middle schools were randomly selected from those of comparable size in demographically similar communities of metropolitan Los Angeles. In terms of school level indicators, student eligibility for free or reduced-price lunch programs ranged from 47% to 87% and all schools qualified for Title I compensatory education funds. Thus, by available indicators, the African American and Latino students who participated in this study were primarily low SES.

All of the data collected on this sample were gathered as part of a written questionnaire administered in classroom settings (see Procedure below). The measures are well-validated instruments that are used widely in school-based research on peer relations and in our own previous research with ethnic minority samples (e.g., Graham & Juvonen, 1998, 2002). For some instruments, subscales were used that most closely captured the constructs of interest.

Self-Report Measures

Self-perceived victimization. Four items from the Peer Victimization Scale (PVS; Neary & Joseph, 1994) and two new items written for this study were used to create a 6-item measure of subjective feelings of victimization. Rather than directly asking students how frequently they get harassed by their peers, we utilized a response format that is designed to reduce social desirability effects (Harter, 1985). For each item, students were presented with two statements separated by the word *But*, with each statement reflecting high or low self-perceived victimization. An example item was: "Some kids are *often* picked on by other kids BUT other kids are *not* picked on by other kids." Students chose one of the two alternatives and then indicated whether the selected alternative is *really true for me* or *sort of true for me*. That creates a 4-point scale for each item. The three other items from the PVS assessed being laughed at, pushed around, and called names. The new items measured whether participants felt that they were gossiped about by others (a form of indirect or relational victimization), and whether their possessions were damaged or stolen by others (direct victimization targeted toward property rather than person). Ratings for the six items were averaged to create a single measure of self-perceived victimization. The scale had good internal consistency ($\alpha = .79$).

Self-esteem. Embedded in the self-perceived victimization measure was the 6-item global self-worth subscale of the Harter Self-Perception Profile for Children (Harter, 1985). For each item, students chose between two statements separated by the word *But*, with each statement reflecting high or low self-worth. An example item was: "Some kids are happy with themselves as a person BUT other kids are often *not* happy with themselves." By rating whether the chosen statement is *really true for me* or *sort of true for me,* a 4-point scale is created. Ratings for the six items were averaged ($\alpha = .77$ for this sample).

Social anxiety. Two subscales from the Social Anxiety Scale for Adolescents (SAS-A, LaGreca & Lopez, 1998) were used to measure fear of negative evaluation (e.g., "I worry about what others think of me") and social avoidance (e.g., "I'm afraid to invite others to do things with me because they might say no"). Each item is rated on a 5-point scale (1 = *not at all* and 5 = *all the time*). Combining the subscales yielded a 12-item measure with good internal consistency ($\alpha = .82$).

Loneliness. A 16-item scale developed by Asher and Wheeler (1985) was used to measure loneliness. Students responded on 5-point scales (1 = *not true at all* through 5 = *always true*) to questions such as "I feel alone" and "I have nobody to talk to." Scores on the 16 items were summed and averaged ($\alpha = .84$).

Depression. Ten items that make up the Short Form of the Children's Depression Inventory (CDI; Kovacs, 1985) were used to assess depressed affect. For each item, respondents were presented with three sentences that describe "how kids might feel" and they chose the sentence that best described how they had been feeling during the past two weeks. A sample item was: "I do most things right"; "I do many things wrong"; "I do everything wrong." Item scores ranged from 0 to 2. Those ratings were summed and averaged ($\alpha = .79$).

Physical symptoms. Students rated how much in the last two weeks they had been bothered by 12 somatic complaints that include headache, upset stomach, poor appetite, and trouble sleeping (1 = *not at all* and 4 = *almost every day*). The 12 items used here were selected from symptom clusters included in other well-established inventories for children and adolescents such as the Children's Somatization Inventory (CSI; Garber, Walker, & Zeman, 1991). Ratings on the 12 items were summed and averaged ($\alpha = .80$).

Peer-Reported Measures

Victim reputation. We used peer nomination procedures to determine which students had reputations as victims. Using a roster that contained the names of all the students in their homeroom, participants were instructed to name up to four students of either gender who fit each of three behavioral descriptions. By restricting the nominations to each homeroom (rather than the larger team or cluster that consisted of up to 120 students), the rosters were more manageable for youth. Two of the behavioral descriptions portrayed physical and verbal harassment (*gets pushed around, gets put down or made fun of by others*). A third description depicted indirect or relational victimization (*other kids spread nasty rumors about them*). The number of nominations each participant received was summed and these scores were standardized within classroom to control for differences in class size.

Social adjustment. Embedded in the peer nomination measure were questions used to measure social adjustment. Respondents nominated up to four classmates whom they *liked to hang out with* and four whom they *did not like to hang out with.* Those nominations measured peer acceptance and rejection, respectively. Finally, participants nominated up to four classmates *who are the coolest kids.* Perceived coolness was judged to capture both popularity and possession of characteristics that are admired among early adolescents. thus, being perceived as cool is not synonymous with acceptance, and in some cases the two measures could elicit disparate nomination patterns (e.g., adolescents might not want to hang out with classmates whom they perceive as most cool). Nomination totals were also summmed for each student and standardized within classroom.

Teacher-Report Measure of Social Adjustment

Homeroom teachers rated the social behavior of participating students using 11 of the original 18 items on the Interpersonal Competence Scale (ICT-T; Cairns, Leung, Gest, & Cairns, 1995). Those items yielded subscales on *internalizing* (3 items, i.e., sad, worries, cries a lot, $\alpha = .59$); *externalizing* (3 items, i.e., starts fights, argues, gets in trouble, $\alpha = .89$) and *popularity* (3 items, i.e., popular with boys (girls), lots of friends, $\alpha = .85$). Each item was presented as a 7-point bipolar scale with anchors unique to that item (e.g., *never sad–always sad, never starts fights–always starts fights, lots of friends–no friends*).

Academic Performance

There were two measures of academic performance: homeroom teacher ratings of school engagement and grade point average (GPA). The degree to which students were perceived to be engaged versus disaffected from school activities was measured with 6 items from the 18-item Teacher Report of Engagement Questionnaire (TREQ; Wellborn & Connell, 1991). An example item was: "In my class this student concentrates on doing his/her work." Ratings were elicited on 4-point scales (1 = *not at all characteristic of this student* and 4 = *very characteristic*). Item scores were summed and averaged ($\alpha = .86$). Data on semester GPA were collected from school records. Grades in academic classes were assigned scores of 0 to 4, with As, Bs, Cs, Ds, and Fs worth 4, 3, 2, 1, and 0 points, respectively. Students' scores were averaged across academic classes to create a single 5-point index of GPA.

Procedure

We recruited 6th grade students from 54 homerooms distributed across eight middle schools. Excluded in each school were self-contained special education classrooms and programs for gifted students. Initially, eligible homeroom teachers were informed about the study. In those classrooms where teachers expressed interest in the study, students took home letters and consent forms in both English and Spanish that explained the study. Only students who returned a signed consent form granting permission were allowed to participate. To increase return rate, students were informed that a raffle would be conducted on the day of data collection for everyone who returned their signed consent forms, with or without parental permission to participate (there was a place on the form to decline participation). In each classroom, two prizes with UCLA logos (e.g., tee-shirts, caps) were raffled at the end of data collection. We achieved an average return rate of 78% (range = 66% to 90% across the eight schools). Of those students who returned a signed consent form, 90% of their parents granted permission for them to participate.

Data were gathered in the Fall of the academic year, once school had been in session for at least two months. Because all of the participating schools organized their 6th graders in teams or clusters, students spent several periods a day with the same classmates and a small number of teachers. Thus by the time of data collection, students knew one another well enough to complete the peer nomination procedures and homeroom teachers knew students well enough to complete the ratings of social behavior and academic engagement.

Questionnaires containing all of the student measures were assembled in booklet form (titled *Middle School Survey*). Before beginning the survey, participants signed a Student Assent form that described our goal to better understand how middle-school students feel about school. They were assured in writing that all responses would be kept confidential and they were encouraged to create "private spaces" at their desks, using their books as well as folders provided by the research team. Graduate student researchers working in pairs administered the questionnaires during an extended block period, since the survey usually required about 1 hour to complete. All instructions and questionnaire items were read aloud by one researcher as students followed along and responded on their own questionnaires. The other researcher circulated around the classroom, helping individual students as needed.

RESULTS

Creation of Victim Subgroups

The first step in the analysis was to create victim groups based on respondents' standardized self-perceived victim scores and peer-nominated victim scores. We followed the procedures used in Graham and Juvonen (1998) to create four groups. Students who were at or above the 70th percentile on both self-ratings and peer nominations were labeled as *true victims* (n = 81, 10% of the sample). *Nonvictims* (*n* = 431, 55% of the sample) were participants whose self- and peer scores fell below the 50th percentile. Students whose self-ratings were at or above the 70th percentile, but whose peer nominations were below the 50th percentile cutoff were classified as *self-identified victims* (*n* = 192, 25% of the sample). Lastly, students who had a reputation for being victims (peer nominations at or above the 70th percentile) but who did not perceive themselves as such (self-ratings below the 50th percentile) were labeled as *peer-identified victims* (*n* = 81, 10% of the sample). Note that more than twice as many participants were classified in the self-identified than in the peer-identified victim group (192 vs. 81). Many youth report experiencing peer harassment in one form or another, whereas fewer individuals have public reputations that are widely endorsed.

Next we examined the victim subgroups by gender and ethnicity of participants. The association between victim status and gender was significant: $\chi^2(3) =$ 42.28, $p < .001$. More than twice as many boys than girls were classified as true victims (57 boys versus 24 girls), whereas the majority of nonvictims were girls (263 girls versus 168 boys). The gender pattern becomes more complex when we consider the groups where peer perceptions and self-perceptions diverged. More boys than girls were classified as peer-identified victims (51 boys versus 31 girls), but more girls than boys embodied the self-identified subgroup (120 girls versus 73 boys). The gender difference was significant in all four victim groups: true victims (z dif = 6.65), self-identified (z dif = 2.80), peer-identified victims (z dif = 4.75), and nonvictims (z dif = 3.07) (all $ps < .05$).

There also was a relationship between victim status and ethnicity, although it was not as strong as that for gender: $\chi^2(3) = 14.23$, $p < .01$. Within group comparisons revealed that the only significant association involved peer-identified victims. Significantly more African Americans (*n* = 52) than Latinos (*n* = 29) had reputations as victims (64% vs 36%, z dif = 5.00, $p < .01$).

In the next set of analyses, we turned to the psychological and social consequences of victim status as defined by self-views and peer appraisals. The psychological adjustment variables (self-esteem, loneliness, anxiety, depression, and physical symptoms), social status variables (peer-nominated acceptance, rejection, and coolness), and teacher rated adjustment variables (internalizing symptoms, externalizing, and popularity) were analyzed in a series of 4 × 2 × 2 (victim group by gender by ethnicity) MANOVAs. Before the analyses, all of the variables were converted into standard scores with a mean of 0 and a standard deviation of 1 to facilitate the interpretation of group differences in measures from multiple informants and with different response scales. Hence, differences among the groups indicate their relative standing within the sample.

Because participants were recruited from eight different schools that varied in ethnic composition, preliminary analyses were conducted on all of the dependent variables with school type (majority Latino, majority African American, mixed ethnicity) as an independent factor. There were no significant main effects on interactions involving school type. The data were, therefore, combined across this variable for all analyses reported here.

Self-Reported Psychological Adjustment

For the five self-report adjustment variables, the multivariate main effect of group was significant, indicating that adjustment varied systematically by victim group status: $F(15, 1946) = 14.55, p < .001$. The top panel of Table 1 shows the means across the four victim groups for each psychological variable, as well as the univariate F-test for that variable. Turning first to the "pure" victim groups in the first and fourth columns, it is evident that true victims reported more psychological maladjustment than did nonvictims. Victims had lower self-esteem than nonvictims and they were more anxious, lonely, depressed, and bothered by physical symptoms. As standard scores ($M = 0, SD = 1$), the

TABLE 1. Mean Differences on the Adjustment and Achievement Variables by Victim Group

	Victim Group				
Variable	True Victims	Self-Ident.	Peer-Ident.	Nonvictims	$F(3, 777)$
Self					
self-esteem	$-.63_a$	$-.40_a$	$.27_b$	$.34_b$	44.92**
anxiety	$.64_a$	$.35_a$	$-.19_b$	$-.31_b$	39.14**
loneliness	$.85_a$	$.20_b$	$.03_b$	$-.34_c$	47.83**
depression	$.84_a$	$.18_b$	$-.28_c$	$-.29_c$	42.36**
symptoms	$.38_a$	$.37_a$	$-.15_b$	$-.20_b$	19.22**
Peer					
acceptance	$-.43_a$	$.07_b$	$-.30_a$	$.22_b$	15.12**
rejection	$.97_a$	$-.28_b$	$.67_c$	$-.29_b$	76.24**
coolness	$-.52_a$	$-.03_b$	$-.09_b$	$.19_b$	13.35**
Teacher					
internalizing	$-.04_a$	$.09_a$	$.06_a$	$-.04_a$	< 1
popularity	$-.58_a$	$.06_b$	$-.30_a$	$.15_b$	16.46**
externalizing	$.68_a$	$-.11_b$	$.74_a$	$-.26_b$	49.62**
Achievement					
engagement	$-.67_a$	$.05_b$	$-.47_a$	$.26_b$	32.67**
GPA	$-.50_a$	$.09_b$	$-.48_a$	$.16_b$	16.29**

Note. Numbers in the table are standard scores. Row means with different subscripts are significantly different at $p < .05$. ** $p < .001$ for the univariate F-tests.

means in Table 1 also can be interpreted in terms of percentiles for this sample (i.e., these scores should not be viewed as clinical cut-offs). Values of 0 are at the 50th percentile; positive scores are above and negative scores are below the 50th percentile. Any score that approaches 1 is at about the 85% percentile and a score that approaches -1 hovers around the 15th percentile. Consider, for example, the loneliness scores of true victims compared to nonvictims. With $M = .85$, true victims lie at the 80th percentile; only about 20% of respondents in this sample would report more loneliness than would true victims. In contrast, with $M = -.34$, nonvictims are at about the 40th percentile; 60% of respondents are predicted to report more loneliness than nonvictims.

The pattern of (mal)adjustment for true victims compared to nonvictims is what we would expect based on previous research. But what about the two groups for whom self- and peer views diverged? For all variables, self-identified and peer-identified victims fell between the two "pure" groups in a systematic way that largely replicated our earlier findings (Graham & Juvonen, 1998). Self-identified victims were more similar to true victims, whereas peer-identified victims consistently resembled nonvictims. For example, students who perceived themselves as victims even when they have no such reputation among peers were just as low in self-esteem and just as anxious and symptomatic as true victims. On the other hand, those students who had reputations as victims were no more depressed, anxious, symptomatic, or low in self-esteem than their nonvictimized counterparts. In sum, the two groups who perceived themselves as victims (true victims and self-identified victims) reported similar levels of maladjustment, whereas the two groups who did not view themselves as victims (peer-identified victims and nonvictims) showed relatively better adjustment.

The pattern displayed in the top panel Table 1 was not influenced by the gender or ethnicity of participants in the different victim groups (i.e., there were no interactions involving gender or ethnicity). However, there was a multivariate main effect of ethnicity, $F(5, 705) = 5.19$, $p < .001$. Independent of victim status and for each variable, Latinos reported more adjustment difficulties than their African American counterparts.

Peer-Reported Social Adjustment

We turn next to social adjustment (acceptance, rejection, coolness) as defined by peer perceptions. Correlational analyses revealed that peer rejection was negatively related to both acceptance ($r = -.23$) and coolness ($r = -.11$). Although acceptance and coolness were positively correlated ($r = .56$), there was still sufficient non-overlap in the meaning of these constructs to examine them separately.

The $4 \times 2 \times 2$ (victim group by gender by ethnicity) MANOVA on the three social adjustment variables documented a significant multivariate effect of victim group, $F(9, 1847) = 20.24$, $p < .001$. Those group effects are displayed in the second panel of Table 1. True victims were less accepted and more rejected than their nonvictimized counterparts. For these variables, however, it was peer-identified rather than self-identified victims who were more similar to true victims. Peer-identified victims were just as disliked as true victims, whereas self-identified victims were just as well liked as nonvictims. Thus, the two groups who had reputations as victims (true victims and peer-identified) had similar levels of social maladjustment, whereas the two groups who did not have such reputations (self-identified victims and nonvictims) showed relatively better social adjustment. For perceived coolness, the group effect was due to the fact that true victims were viewed as less cool than were the other three groups who did not differ significantly from one another.

There were more gender and ethnicity effects in these analyses, which highlights some of the determinants of social status among middle-school students. Girls were more accepted than boys and they were less rejected: multivariate $F(3, 759) = 4.02$, $p < .01$. African American students were more disliked than Latinos, but they were also perceived as more cool: multivariate $F(3, 759) = 5.68$, $p < .001$. Thus students tended to dislike some classmates whom they viewed as most cool. A 3-way interaction for coolness indicated that African American boys who peers considered to be victims were judged to be especially cool: $F(3, 761) = 2.84$, p < .05.

Teacher-Perceived Social Adjustment

Teachers provide an independent informant source because their perceptions did not enter into the creation of victim groups. For teacher perceptions, there was a multivariate main effect of victim group, $F(9, 1789) = 13.38$, $p < .001$ (see third panel of Table 1). Univariate ANOVAs revealed no effects of victim group for teacher-perceived internalizing symptoms. Teachers perceived nonvictims and self-identified victims to be more popular than true and peer-identified victims, but the opposite was true for the more negative externalizing (aggressive) behavior. In many ways, therefore, the teacher judgments were consistent with those of peers. Peer-identified victims were judged as poorly on these social outcomes as true victims, while self-identified victims fared as well as nonvictims.

There were also gender and ethnicity main effects for teacher judgments. The multivariate gender effect revealed that girls were viewed as more popular and less aggressive than boys: $F(3, 735) = 7.01$, $p < .001$. The multivariate ethnicity effect showed that African Americans were judged as more popular than

Latinos, but also as more aggressive: $F(3, 735) = 11.98$, $p < .001$. The multivariate group $\times$ gender $\times$ ethnicity interaction was explained by the fact that the most aggressive students in the teacher's eyes were African American boys who were identified by their peers as victims: $F(9, 1789) = 2.05, p < .05$.

Academic Achievement

To examine school outcomes, we analyzed teacher ratings of academic engagement and students' semester GPA in separate $4 \times 2 \times 2$ ANOVAs (bottom panel of Table 1). For academic engagement there were main effects of victim group, $F(3, 733) = 32.67$, gender, $F(1, 733) = 9.57$; and ethnicity, $F(1, 733) = 32.13$ (all $ps < .01$). Consistent with the psychological and social variables, true victims were rated as less engaged than nonvictims. However, peer-identified victims resembled true victims in being relatively disengaged, whereas self-identified victims were akin to nonvictims in being perceived as relatively engaged. Furthermore, girls were rated more positively than boys and Latinos were judged more positively than African Americans.

There was an identical pattern to the data for actual grades: $Fs = 16.29$, 15.84, and 29.49 for the victim group, gender, and ethnicity main effects (all $ps <$ .001). The academic advantage that nonvictims enjoyed was shared by self-identified victims, while the relatively poor achievement of true victims also was characteristic of peer-identified victims. The gender and ethnicity main effects indicated that girls had better grades than boys and Latinos did significantly better than African Americans. None of the interactions were significant for either achievement variable.

Relations Between Variables: Predicting GPA

We know from the group analyses that being the victim of peer harassment was related to academic GPA. But what role might the psychological and social adjustment play in this relation? We hypothesized that the effect of self- and peer-perceived victimization on academic achievement would be largely explained by the adjustment outcomes. Thus, for example, perceiving oneself as a victim undermines school performance because of the psychological costs (e.g., depression, anxiety) that often accompany those self-views. Psychological maladjustment, in other words, was thought to be the more proximal determinant of poor grades. Similarly, having a reputation as a victim predicts low achievement because such children suffer the added burden of being rejected by their peers.

Path analysis was used to examine the hypothesized predictors of GPA. In path analysis the researcher can specify a set of relationships between variables and then test whether the specified model adequately fits the data. One index of model fit is the χ^2 statistic. A nonsignificant χ^2 (i.e., no difference between the tested model and the actual data) indicates a good fit.

The best fitting model of the relations between variables is shown in Figure 1: $\chi^2(4) = 4.81$, *ns*. Note first that self- and peer-perceived victimization are only modestly correlated ($r = .19$), which means that there was little overlap between self-views and peer views, as we have emphasized in this article. Once these perceptions are activated, the model proposes two relatively independent sequences, with the upper pathway depicting the psychological processes affecting school achievement and the lower sequence portraying social mechanisms. The psychological adjustment variables were averaged to create a single index (average $r = .42$) and peer rejection was used as the social adjustment variable. In the first sequence, self-perceived victimization predicted psychological maladjustment ($\beta = .50$) and maladjustment, in turn, predicted low achievement ($\beta = -.18$). In the second sequence, victim reputation resulted in peer rejection ($\beta = .56$) and rejection was then related to diminished performance ($\beta = -.27$). Having a reputation as a victim was also moderately related to maladjustment ($\beta = .13$), which suggests that students are aware of how they are perceived in the eyes of others and that awareness influenced their own self-views.

DISCUSSION

Being a victim of peer harassment places students at risk for many kinds of adjustment difficulties. Some of those adjustment challenges relate to self-appraisals, whereas others can be linked to the social context and one's reputation among teachers and peers. Still other consequences involve academic outcomes such as perceived engagement and grades. The findings presented here suggest that particular types of victims are vulnerable to specific kinds of

FIGURE 1. Path Analysis of Relations Between Victimization, Adjustment, and Academic Achievement.

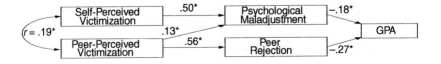

maladjustment. Both self-reports of harassment experiences and peer reports of victim status are necessary to capture the full range of victim subgroups and the unique challenges of each.

"True" Victims: When Self- and Peer Views Converge

The best evidence for the negative consequences of peer harassment was seen in the group who felt like victims and had that reputation among peers. For every adjustment variable examined in this research, there were reliable differences between true victims and nonvictims, with the difference always favoring nonvictims. These findings replicate prior studies and underscore the fact that peer victimization cuts across race, SES, and different school contexts.

Self-Identified and Peer-Identified Victims: When Self- and Peer Views Diverge

For purposes of identification, the most challenging findings emerged for the victimized students for whom self- and peer perceptions were discrepant. On the self-report indexes (depression, anxiety, etc.) self-identified victims were consistently more similar to true victims, whereas peer-identified victims responded more like nonvictims. But on the peer-focused indexes (acceptance and rejection) peer-identified victims were just as rejected as true victims, whereas self-identified victims were as accepted as nonvictims. Had we relied only on self-reports we might wrongly have concluded that victimization is not associated with peer rejection. Had we relied only on peer reports, we might have been similarly misguided in concluding that victimization is not related to negative feelings about the self. In the path analysis, *both* maladjustment and peer rejection were risk factors for academic problems.

Because the two victim groups are linked to different risk factors, one might wonder whether there is any reason to think that one group is more vulnerable than the other. Concerning self-identified victims, a large body of clinical research has documented the short- and long-term effects of adolescent depression, anxiety, and low self-worth (Steinberg & Morris, 2001). That research reports greater mental health challenges for adolescent girls, which is consistent with our finding that the majority of self-identified victims were girls. Thus there is reason to be concerned about self-identified victims if they react to their plight by turning inward. In previous research, we found that self-identified victims, like true victims, were more likely to blame themselves for being picked on by others (Graham & Juvonen, 1998). They were more willing to endorse such statements as "It must be *me*" or "Why do *I* always get into these situations?" Self-blame then accounted for most of their negative feelings about themselves. Equally of concern is that disparaging self-views and depressed affect may go unnoticed by teachers. Recall that teachers in this study did not differentiate among victim groups (including nonvictims) when they rated the degree to which students were sad, worried, or tearful–the set of variables that we labeled as internalizing symptoms (see Table 1).

On the other hand, self-identified victims enjoyed widespread acceptance among their peers and their teachers perceived them to be popular and socially competent. As a group, they also were doing reasonably well in school. For some self-identified victims, it could be that the peer support and teacher approval were protective factors that lessened the impact of victim status.

Peer-identified victims, who were primarily boys and primarily African American, had quite a different risk profile. They did not view themselves as victims and they did not report disparaging self-views. Perhaps the incidents that peers perceive as harassment were not subjectively experienced in that way by these youth who may also be reluctant to report that they are victimized–an admission that implies that they are unable to defend themselves. Several studies have suggested that African American adolescent boys sometimes exhibit exaggerated behavioral and emotional toughness, called male *bravado,* as a way of coping with negative experiences (e.g., Cunningham, 1999). Such coping styles may contribute to peer perceptions of this particular victim group as "cool" and an attraction to these boys who enjoy a particular kind of notoriety. Yet these peer-identified victims were also disliked by some of their classmates. The reputations of peer-identified victims were quite public in that teachers shared the negative views of peers. These students also were doing as poorly in school as true victims. Therefore, the benefits of positive self-views and some notoriety among peers did not offset the risks associated with victim reputation.

Limitations of the Current Study

Our sample of young Latino and African-American adolescents is a unique one and thus we do not know how well the findings regarding the two divergent victim groups will replicate across other samples. Our findings may have been influenced not only by the demographics of the participants (ethnicity, SES, community characteristics) but also the particular schools contexts in which they reside. We did not uncover any school effects based on one contextual variable–the ethnic composition of schools–but other classroom and school effects warrant attention in future research. New statistical methods, such as hierarchical linear modeling (HLM), provide appropriate tools to examine such questions. Finally, we acknowledge that our cross-sectional data do not permit us to make causal inferences about the consequences of victimization. Yet the findings do provide a framework for testing the directionality of effects with longitudinal data from the larger project.

Implications for Assessment and Intervention

We believe that enriching the study of peer harassment to distinguish victims for whom self- and peer-perceptions diverge has important implications for both assessment and intervention. If identification procedures rely primarily on reports of others, such as reputation among peers or teacher impressions, then we would have missed 192 students in our sample (self-identified victims) who felt vulnerable and victimized but did not have that reputation among their peers. Because youth in general are reluctant to seek help for peer harassment, and because these self-identified youth enjoyed a level of peer acceptance similar to nonvictims, it is unlikely that their adjustment problems would have been detected in the absence of self-report data.

What intervention strategies would be most helpful to self-identified victims given their particular vulnerabilities? One area of vulnerability might be their tendency to think that their own plight is unique (i.e., "I am the only one who gets picked on"). Preliminary evidence to support that assertion comes from a study in which children kept a daily diary of specific peer harassment incidents (Nishina & Juvonen, 2002). The analyses across a 2-week period showed that the frequency of harassment incidents predicted negative self-views only for those children who never reported seeing other students getting picked on. Hence, the self-identified group might benefit from intervention approaches where the pervasiveness of the problem is acknowledged (i.e., "It's *not* just me"). But that strategy alone would not reduce anxiety or fear associated with repeated harassment. Teaching behavioral skills that allow youth to effectively respond to harassment episodes (e.g., leaving the situation before it escalates, staying with a group) would be likely to alleviate some of their anxieties. Both of these intervention strategies (changing perceptions of one's plight as unique and acquiring a behavioral repertoire to ward off victimization) can be accomplished by using a systemic, whole-school approach where all students are involved (Olweus, 1993).

Just as the self-identified victim group is likely to remain undiagnosed unless self-report instruments are used, the peer-identified victims would go undetected if the assessment relies only on self-reports. Because victims are highly likely to be rejected, the omission of the peer-identified group would constitute a serious oversight, given how much we know about peer rejection as a risk factor for many negative outcomes (e.g., Kupersmidt, Coie, & Dodge, 1990). Had we not included peer reports of victimization in the current sample, we would have missed the 81 students who had only social reputations as victims.

One of the challenges of intervention with peer-identified victims has to do with their level of awareness. It is not clear whether these youth knowingly refuse to admit that they get picked on by peers or whether they are simply unaware of their problems. Some degree of positive illusion may be adaptive (Taylor & Brown, 1988). But illusory beliefs are detrimental when they interfere with a person's ability to understand the effects of their behavior on others. In our study, some of the peer-identified victims (particularly African American boys) were rated by their teachers as having externalizing problems. In those cases, it is likely that these youth get harassed because they (are perceived to) provoke others. Some of the known strategies for helping aggressive youth to better handle peer provocation might, therefore, be useful for children such as peer-identified victims. For example, teaching aggressive students to recognize when provocations are accidental rather than intended has proven to be an effective intervention (Hudley & Graham, 1993; Graham, Taylor, & Hudley, 2002). Conflict mediation as part of an anti-bullying prevention approach also is recommended. Such approaches typically involve analyses of specific incidents in terms of "who did what and when." Those activities provide helpful feedback to youth about how they may have contributed to a particular harassment incident and what they could do differently in the future.

By comparing self-reports and peer reports of victimization, we have demonstrated that identifying the targets of peer harassment is complex. We are not advocating one method over another, nor are we proposing that school mental health professionals should conduct routine grade-wide screenings to identify victimized youth. Rather, we wanted to point out that different types of victims might be identified with each method and that findings of studies can vary depending on the type of assessment used. As long as the presence of peer harassment shapes the culture and climate of schools, it is important that professional staff be aware that the subjective experience of feeling victimized and the reputation as a victim in the eyes of others are distinct, albeit partly overlapping, phenomena. To our knowledge, whether agreement between different informants would change as a function of certain school-wide prevention programs has not been tested.

Beyond Victimization

With a large multiethnic sample, we would feel remiss if we did not call attention to some of the ethnicity main effects that emerged in the analysis independent of victim status. Those findings remind us of the broader social context in which adolescents of color live and the multiple challenges that they often face. On the psychological adjustment variables, Latinos reported more nega- tive feelings (e.g., depression, anxiety) than did African Americans. The ma- jority of Latino students in our sample were children of immigrants and they attended schools that had large enrollments of Latinos with similar immigrant histories. Much has been written about the adjustment challenges of these sec- ond generation youth and of the need for schools to be particularly sensitive to their psychosocial needs (Portes, 1996; Suarez-Orozco & Suarez- Orozco, 2001). On the social variables, African American boys were judged in a more negative light (e.g., more rejected by peers, displaying externalizing problems) than were Latinos. Much also has been written about the adjustment chal- lenges of African American males and the stress of coping with negative eval- uations of their group (e.g., Graham, Taylor, & Hudley, 1998; Spencer, Cunningham, & Swanson, 1995). Both sets of problems that we highlight–the psychological and the social–are risk factors for poor school achievement. Be- ing an adolescent of color *and* a victim of peer harassment only magnifies that risk.

REFERENCES

Asher, S., & Wheeler, V. (1985). Children's loneliness: A comparison of neglected and rejected peer status. *Journal of Consulting and Clinical Psychology, 53,* 500-505.
Astor, R., Meyer, H., & Behre, W. (1999). Unowned places and times: Maps and interviews about violence in high schools. *American Educational Research Journal, 36,* 3-42.
Cairns, R., Leung, M., Gest, S., & Cairns, B. (1995). A brief method for assessing so- cial development: Structure, reliability, stability, and developmental validity of the Interpersonal Competence Scale. *Behavioral Research and Therapy, 33,* 725-736.
Crick, N., & Grotpeter, J. (1996). Children's treatment by peers: Victims of relational and overt aggression. *Development and Psychopathology, 8,* 367-380.
Cunningham, M. (1999). African American adolescent males' perceptions of their community resources and constraints: A longitudinal analysis. *Journal of Commu- nity Psychology, 27,* 569-588.
Garber, J., Walker, L., & Zeman, J. (1991). Somatization symptoms in a community sample of children and adolescents: Further validation of the Children's Somatization Inventory. *Psychological Assessment, 3,* 588-595.
Graham, S., & Juvonen, J. (1998). Self-blame and peer victimization in middle school: An attributional analysis. *Developmental Psychology, 34,* 587-599.
Graham, S., & Juvonen, J. (2002). Ethnicity, peer harassment, and adjustment in mid- dle school: An exploratory study. *Journal of Early Adolescence, 22,* 173-199.
Graham, S., Taylor, A., & Hudley, C. (1998). Exploring achievement values among ethnic minority early adolescents. *Journal of Educational Psychology, 90,* 606-620.
Graham, S., Taylor, A., & Hudley, C. (2002). *A social skills and academic motivation intervention for at-risk African American boys.* Manuscript submitted for publica- tion.

Harter, S. (1985). *The self-perception scale profile for children: Revision of the Perceived Competence Scale for Children manual.* Denver, CO: University of Denver Press.

Hudley, C., & Graham, S. (1993). An attributional intervention to reduce peer-directed aggression among African American boys. *Child Development, 64,* 124-138.

Hymel, S., Wagner, E., & Butler, L. (1990). Reputational bias: View from the peer group. In S. Asher & J. Coie (Eds.), *Peer rejection in childhood* (pp. 156-186). New York: Cambridge University Press.

Juvonen, J., Nishina, A., & Graham, S. (2000). Peer harassment, psychological well-being, and school adjustment in early adolescence. *Journal of Educational Psychology, 92,* 349-359.

Juvonen, S., Nishina, A., & Graham, S. (2001). Self-views versus peer perceptions of victimization among early adolescents. In J. Juvonen and S. Graham (Eds.), *Peer harassment in school: The plight of the vulnerable and victimized* (pp. 105-124). New York: Guilford Press.

Kochenderfer, B., & Ladd, G. (1996). Peer victimization: Cause or consequence of children's school adjustment difficulties? *Child Development, 67,* 1305-1317.

Kovacs, M. (1985). The Children's Depression Inventory: A self-rated depression scale for school-aged youngsters. *Psychopharmacology Bulletin, 21,* 995-998.

Kupersmidt, J. B., Coie, J. D., & Dodge, K. A. (1990). The role of poor peer relationships in the development of disorder. In S. R. Asher & J. D. Coie (Eds.), *Peer rejection in childhood* (pp. 274-305). New York: Cambridge University Press.

La Greca, A., & Lopez, N. (1998). Social anxiety among adolescents: Linkages with peer relations and friendships. *Journal of Abnormal Child Psychology, 26,* 83-94.

Nansel, T., Overpeck, M., Pilla, R., Ruan, W., Simons-Morton, B., & Scheidt, P. (2001). Bullying behavior among US youth. Prevalence and association with psychological adjustment. *Journal of the American Medical Association, 285,* 2094-2100.

Neary, A., & Joseph, S. (1994). Peer victimization and its relationship to self-concept and depression among schoolgirls. *Personality and Individual Differences, 16,* 183-186.

Nishina, A. & Juvonen, J. (2002). *Daily reports of negative affect and peer harassment in middle school.* Manuscript submitted for publication.

Olweus, D. (1993). *Bullying at school: What we know and what we can do.* Oxford, UK: Blackwell.

Pelligrini, A. (2001). Sampling instances of victimization in middle school: A methodological comparison. In J. Juvonen and S. Graham (Eds.), *Peer harassment in school: The plight of the vulnerable and victimized* (pp. 124-144). New York: Guilford Press.

Portes, A. (Ed.). (1996). *The new second generation.* New York: The Russell Sage Foundation.

Schuster, B. (1996). Rejection, exclusion, and harassment at work and in schools: An integration of results from research on mobbing, bullying, and peer rejection. *European Psychologist, 1,* 293-317.

Spencer, M., Cunningham, M., & Swanson, D. (1995). Identity as coping: Adolescent African American males' adaptive responses to high-risk environments. In H. Blue,

E. Griffith, & H. Harris (Eds.), *Racial and ethnic identity: Psychological development and creative expression* (pp. 31-52). New York: Routledge Publishers.

Steinberg, L., & Morris, A. (2001). Adolescent development. *Annual Review of Psychology, Vol. 52* (pp. 83-110). Palo Alto, CA: Annual Reviews.

Suarez-Orozco, C., & Suarez-Orozco, M. (2001). *Children of immigration.* Cambridge, MA: Harvard University Press.

Taylor, S., & Brown, J. (1988). Illusion and well-being: A social psychological perspective on mental health. *Psychological Bulletin, 103,* 193-210.

Wellborn, J., & Connell, J. (1991), *Students' achievement relevant ions in the classroom. A self-report measure of student motivation.* Unpublished manuscript. University of Rochester.

Developmental Trajectories of Victimization: Identifying Risk and Protective Factors

Suzanne Goldbaum
Wendy M. Craig

Queen's University

Debra Pepler
Jennifer Connolly

York University

SUMMARY. Using a modified version of Olweus' victimization (Student Questionnaire, 1993) scale, 1,241 children in Grades 5 to 7 from diverse socioeconomic neighborhoods were classified into four distinct trajectories of victimization: non-victims, late onset victims, stable victims, and desisters. MANCOVAS investigated how changes in victimization across different trajectories corresponded to variations in intra- and interpersonal functioning. Risk factors including anxiety and low friendship quality lead to subsequent victimization and these problems in-

---

Address correspondence to: Wendy M. Craig, Department of Psychology, Queen's University, Kingston, Ontario, Canada K7L 3N6 (E-mail: craigw@psyc.queensu.ca).

This research was supported by grants from the Ontario Mental Health Foundation and The National Health Research and Development Program.

The authors would like to acknowledge the schools and students who participated in this research study.

[Haworth co-indexing entry note]: "Developmental Trajectories of Victimization: Identifying Risk and Protective Factors." Goldbaum, Suzanne et al. Co-published simultaneously in *Journal of Applied School Psychology* (The Haworth Press, Inc.) Vol. 19, No. 2, 2003, pp. 139-156; and: *Bullying, Peer Harassment, and Victimization in the Schools: The Next Generation of Prevention* (ed: Maurice J. Elias, and Joseph E. Zins) The Haworth Press, Inc., 2003, pp. 139-156. Single or multiple copies of this article are available for a fee from The Haworth Document Delivery Service [1-800-HAWORTH, 9:00 a.m. - 5:00 p.m. (EST). E-mail address: docdelivery@haworthpress.com].

10.1300/J008v19n02_09

creased with continued victimization. Engaging in fewer aggressive behaviors, having high quality friendships, and experiencing low levels of anxiety were identified as factors that protect adolescents from future victimization. The discussion focuses on the possible mechanisms contributing to the maintenance or changes in levels of victimization, and how interventions can reduce peer victimization in schools. *[Article copies available for a fee from The Haworth Document Delivery Service: 1-800-HAWORTH. E-mail address: <docdelivery@haworthpress.com> Website: <http://www.HaworthPress. com> © 2003 by The Haworth Press, Inc. All rights reserved.]*

KEYWORDS. Trajectories, victimization, risk factors, protective mechanisms, intervention

Peer bullying and victimization occur frequently among children. According to Olweus (1991), victims of bullying are exposed to repeated acts over time by someone in a position of more power, that cause them marked distress. Prevalence rates of victimization are consistent across different countries (Farrington, 1993). In Canada, researchers have found that 49% of students reported being bullied at least once or twice during the term, when different forms of bullying (e.g., verbal and physical) are considered together. Eight percent of children report being bullied regularly, at least once a week (Charach, Pepler, & Ziegler, 1995). Repeated victimization is an impediment to children's healthy social and emotional development. Adjustment problems such as depression and low self-esteem are associated with victimization (Craig, 1998). This form of harassment also is related to aggression; running away from home; alcohol and drug use; dropping out of school; and committing suicide (Olweus, 1992). Finally, research suggests that childhood victimization strongly predicts later behavior adjustment and adult disturbance (Parker & Asher, 1987).

Despite the general consensus regarding prevalence rates of victimization, the predominant use of cross-sectional designs precludes investigations of the stability of victimization and how effects of victimization change over time. The present study provides insight by using a longitudinal research design and a group-based approach that identifies victimization trajectories (Nagin, 1999). In addition, differences among participants in the victimization trajectories were investigated in order to identify risk and protective factors associated with different developmental patterns of victimization. Because of the cumulative effects of risk factors over time, it was predicted that the longer an individual is victimized, the more aversive the associated psychological outcomes. In addition to the duration of victimization, other individual and peer factors may act as risk or protection for the negative outcomes associated with victimization. Identification of these factors will provide direction for the development of prevention and intervention programs aimed at reducing victimization and promoting healthy development.

INTRAPERSONAL CHARACTERISTICS OF VICTIMS

Previous research identifies a number of risk factors that are associated with victimization, including internalizing problems such as anxiety, depression, loneliness, somatization, and low self-esteem (Boulton & Underwood, 1992; Craig, 1998). Since previous studies were primarily cross-sectional, the ways in which these variables changed relative to changes in victimization is not clear. Thus, investigations are needed to determine if these intrapersonal problems preceded, are maintained, or were a consequence of victimization. Our longitudinal analysis and identification of trajectories may facilitate this understanding.

Interpersonal Factors Associated with Victimization

Aggressive behaviors also are commonly associated with victimization, though as with intrapersonal factors, the possible sequential relationship between aggression and victimization has not been investigated. Some children who are victimized are passive and do not overtly respond to their abuse, while others react to attacks in an aggressive manner (Pellegrini, 1998). This second category of victims is labeled victim/bullies, and these individuals are considered to be at increased risk for internalizing and externalizing disorders (Austin & Joseph, 1996), as well as the most severe rejection among peers (Pellegrini, 1998). Kochenderfer and Ladd (1997) found that children who 'fought back' were more likely to have a stable pattern of victimization. Similarly, compared to bullies and victims, victim/bullies were particularly at risk for prolonged involvement in bullying interactions (Kumpulainen, Raesaenen, & Henttonen, 1999). These studies highlight the importance of understanding how aggression relates to victimization and how they change together over time. The present study assessed changes in aggressive and bullying behavior across different trajectories of victimization.

In addition to aggressive behavior, interpersonal factors such as friendships and peer group status also are associated with victimization. Children in a mutual best friendship or popular children with more friends are less likely than rejected children with fewer friends to report internalizing and externalizing behaviors otherwise predicted by victimization (Hodges, Boivin, Vitaro, & Bukowski, 1999; Hodges, Malone, & Perry, 1997). The lack of a supportive network of friends put children at considerably more risk than children with an adequate support system. Salmivalli, Huttunen, and Lagerspetz (1997) concluded that victims and defenders had the smallest peer networks and of the children who did not belong to any peer network, almost half were victims. If victims do not belong to a peer group, they may not benefit from peer group socialization experiences that are normally associated with the peer group (i.e., protection), and that are a requisite for healthy social development.

While previous research indicates that the number of friends children have, their popularity, as well as likeability correlate with victim status (Hodges et al., 1997), it is possible that friendship quality also plays a role in victimization. Since victims do report having some friends, it may be that lower quality relationships account for their lack of protection from friends. Friendship qualities such as trust and affection are important in developing intimate relationships. If high levels of these friendship qualities do not characterize victims' friendships, victims may not effectively communicate their distress and seek support and protection from their friends. The present study examined the quality of participants' friendships as well as their social competence.

In summary, this study had three goals: To identify (1) the trajectories of victimization; (2) intra- and interpersonal risk and protective factors associated with victimization; and (3) the consequences associated with stable victimization.

METHOD

Participants

Participants were 635 boys and 606 girls enrolled in seven schools in a large urban Canadian city. At the beginning of the study, participants were in Grade 5 (N = 313), Grade 6 (N = 376) and Grade 7 (N = 552). Previous research suggests that students in these grades report similar patterns of victimization over time (Goldbaum & Craig, 2001), and therefore grade differences were not examined. There were three test administrations (Time 1 = fall year 1; Time 2 = spring year 1; Time 3 = fall year 2), and participants' ages ranged between 9 and 14. There was a 5% attrition rate. Schools represented diverse socioeconomic backgrounds. Both parent and child consent were obtained, with an overall participation rate of 84%. Seventy-seven percent and 72% of fathers and mothers, respectively, were university graduates; 17% and 22%, respectively, were high school or community college graduates; and 5% of fathers and mothers did not graduate from high school. The majority of participants identified themselves as European Canadian (74%); 4% as African or Caribbean-Canadian; 10% as Native or Asian Canadian; and 11% identified their race in other ways. Seventy-five percent of participants lived with both parents; 13% lived with one natural parent; 12% of participants had other family configurations.

Measures

Victimization. A modified *Bully/Victim Questionnaire* (Olweus, 1993) derived victimization scores from two items, "About how many times have you been bullied in the last five days at school?" and "How often have you been bullied at school since the beginning of the school year?" Examples of bullying are provided (i.e., physical and verbal). Students responded on a five-point scale, with '0' meaning 'it hasn't happened,' and '4' representing 'several times a week' for the first question, and 'five or more times' for the second question. Scores were standardized and used for group formation. Cronbach alphas for the three test administrations ranged from 0.80 to 0.85.

A modified version of the *Conflict Tactics Scale* (Straus, 1979) evaluated direct physical victimization. Respondents indicated on an 11-point scale how often each of six actions had occurred to them since the beginning of the school year, where higher numbers represent higher frequencies of events. Items were specific to close friends, peers, and romantic partners. Cronbach alphas ranged from 0.60 to 0.72.

Internalizing problems. The *Child Behavior Checklist-Youth Self-Report* (CBCL-YSR) (Achenbach, 1991) assessed internalizing dimensions, including anxiety/depression, somatization, and withdrawal. Participants responded on a scale ranging from '0' to '2' ('Not true,' 'Somewhat or sometimes true,' or 'Very true or often true') indicating how frequently each item occurred in the past two months. Higher scores represented more internalizing problems. Fourteen items comprised the anxiety/depression subscale which revealed alphas ranging from 0.86 to 0.88. Somatization was a reliable nine-item scale and alphas ranged from 0.77 to 0.80. The withdrawal subscale comprised seven items, and alphas ranged from 0.67 to 0.71.

Social self-competence. A modified version of Harter's *Perceived Competence Scale for Children* (1982) assessed participants' perceived social competence using a structured alternative format. Children indicated which description best described them and then chose whether it was 'really' or 'sort of' true. Each item was scored from 1 to 4, where a score of 1 reflects low perceived competence and 4 indicates high perceived competence. Only the 5-item social competence subscale was used in the present study. Alphas ranged from 0.77 to 0.80.

Peer relations. A modification of the *People in My Life Scale* (Armsden & Greenberg, 1987; Furman & Buhrmester, 1995) assessed children's relationships with friends. Participants rated on a five-point scale (ranging from 'Almost never or never true' to 'Almost always or always true'), high numbers representing higher levels of friendship qualities. Eleven items assessed trust (alphas from 0.89 to 0.93), four questions measured communication (alphas from 0.85 to 0.88), four items assessed alienation (alphas from 0.58 to 0.72), affection had two questions (alphas from 0.68 to 0.76), three items measured commitment (alphas from 0.75 to 0.79), and three items assessed intimacy (alphas from 0.80 to 0.87) in participants' friendships.

Aggression. Achenbach's *YSR* (1991) measured self-reported aggression. The 19 questions demonstrated sufficient reliability (alphas ranged from 0.71 to 0.88).

Bullying. A modified *Bully/Victim Questionnaire* (Olweus, 1993), as described for victimization, was used to derive a bullying scale and demonstrated acceptable reliabilities (alphas ranged from 0.78 to 0.81). Bullying was measured with two items, each assessed on a five-point scale, where higher numbers represented more bullying.

RESULTS

Group formation. Previous studies categorizing children as victims employed arbitrary cut-off points in defining victimization group membership (Boulton & Underwood, 1992). While these classifications may be theoretically reasonable, they do not necessarily exist naturally, and may be based on potentially misleading categorizations. Advancements in methodology for examining individuals' developmental trajectories provide researchers with the ability to transcend the use of these traditional categorization procedures. Another advantage of the new technique (TRAJ) is that in contrast to hierarchical and latent growth curve modeling, it makes no assumptions regarding a continuous distribution of trajectories (Nagin & Tremblay, 1999) and this method identifies the existing differences among groups.

Results of the trajectory analyses indicated that a four-group model best represents how participants' levels of victimization change over time. Analyses comparing competing trajectories of victimization are described elsewhere (see Goldbaum & Craig, 2001). The following four groups were identified: non-victims reported consistently low levels of victimization; desisters started with high levels of victimization which decreased over time; late onset victims reported increasing levels of victimization; and stable victims reported consistently high levels of victimization. Participants were assigned a probability for group membership for each trajectory that assessed how closely they represent each identified group (see Table 1). Whereas victimization changed over time for desisters and late onset victims (and slightly for stable victims), non-victims did not report changes in victimization over time (Figure 1).

A MANOVA testing an independent self-reported measure of physical victimization revealed a significant time by group interaction, multivariate F (3, 966) = 13.33, $p < .001$, attesting to the validity of the groups. Participants' changing levels of physical victimization corresponded to the shape of their respective groups' victimization trajectories: increases and decreases in physical victimization coincided with increases and decreases in the measure of victimization used to form the trajectories. The group of non-victims consistently reported low levels of physical victimization, while stable victims consistently reported the highest levels.

GROUP DIFFERENCES

To investigate differences among the four groups over time, repeated measures MANCOVAs were performed. Because of the small number of participants classified as stable victims, desisters, and late onset victims, sex was entered as a covariate. A chi square analysis indicated that boys and girls were equally represented in the groups.

Intrapersonal Factors

Internalizing problems. Results showed a significant time by group interaction, multivariate F (18, 2511) = 2.65, $p < .001$, with associated univariate effects of anxiety, F (6, 1680) = 5.54, $p < .001$, and withdrawal, F (6, 1680) = 4.72, $p < .001$ (see Table 2 for means and standard deviations). Post hoc analy-

TABLE 1. Mean Probabilities (and Standard Deviations) of Group Membership and Number of Participants in Each Group

	Non-victims	Desisters	Late onset victims	Stable victims
Probabilities	.99 (.04)	.95 (.11)	.95 (.11)	.96 (.10)
Males	546	44	33	12
Females	543	32	23	8

FIGURE 1. Trajectories of Victimization

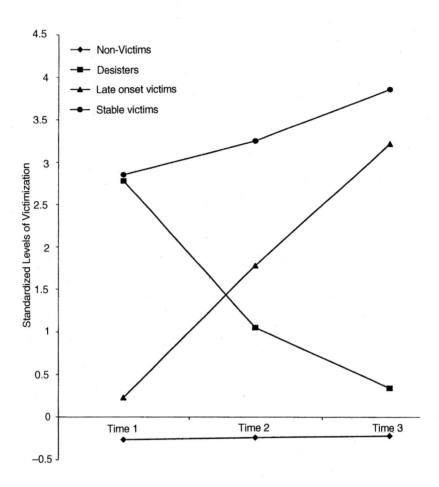

ses indicated that non-victims always reported the lowest levels of anxiety. Late onset victims reported less anxiety than stable victims at Times 1 and 2, though by Time 3, their anxiety was comparable to stable victims, and their anxiety was higher than the desisters'. Desisters initially did not report less anxiety than stable victims, though by Times 2 and 3, desisters reported less anxiety than did stable and late onset victims. Late onset victims initially reported similar levels of anxiety to desisters (which was high at Time 1), suggesting that high levels of anxiety preceded increases in victimization. Planned contrasts examined whether any group reported significant changes in anxiety

TABLE 2. Means (and Standard Deviations) for Internalizing Problems

Time of testing	Non-victims	Desisters	Late onset victims	Stable victims
		Anxiety		
1	0.36 (0.31)[a]	0.73 (0.36)[b]	0.70 (0.47)[b]	0.92 (0.59)[c]
2	0.30 (0.33)[a]	0.51 (0.36)[b]	0.63 (0.60)[b]	1.00 (0.60)[c]
3	0.29 (0.33)[a]	0.44 (0.29)[b]	0.76 (0.54)[c]	0.94 (0.56)[c]
		Withdrawal		
1	0.37 (0.30)[a]	0.61 (0.34)[b]	0.55 (0.40)[b]	0.73 (0.49)[b]
2	0.32 (0.31)[a]	0.44 (0.39)[b]	0.47 (0.41)[b]	0.87 (0.54)[c]
3	0.30 (0.30)[a]	0.34 (0.32)[a]	0.56 (0.45)[b]	0.62 (0.44)[b]

Note. Means in the same row that do not share subscripts differ at $p < .05$.

over time. Desisters reported decreasing levels of anxiety from Time 1 to Time 3, $F (1, 1680) = 24.92, p < .001$.

At Times 1 and 2 non-victims reported less withdrawal than did all other participants. At Time 3, however, desisters reported similar levels of withdrawal to non-victims. At Time 2, stable victims reported the highest levels of withdrawal, though by Time 3, late onset victims reported similar levels of withdrawal to stable victims. Desisters reported decreasing levels of withdrawal from Time 1 to Time 3, $F (1, 1680) = 22.00, p < .001$.

The MANCOVA also revealed a main effect of group, multivariate $F (9, 2520) = 14.80, p < .001$, with associated univariate effects for anxiety, $F (3, 840) = 43.71, p < .001$; withdrawal, $F (3, 840) = 17.36, p < .001$; and somatization, $F (3, 840) = 19.50, p < .001$. For all internalizing problems, non-victims and stable victims were significantly different from each of the other groups, reporting the lowest and highest scores, respectively.

Interpersonal Factors

Social self-competence and friendships. In the MANCOVA assessing group differences in social self-competence and friendship quality, there was a significant time by group interaction, multivariate $F (42, 2139) = 1.71, p < .01$, with associated univariate effects on social self-competence, $F (6, 1448) = 4.21, p < .001$; trust, $F (6, 1448) = 4.03, p < .01$; and affection, $F (6, 1448) = 3.65, p < .01$ (see Table 3). Non-victims initially reported higher levels of social self-competence than did desisters or stable victims; and by Times 2 and 3, they reported the highest levels of social self-competence. At Times 1 and 2 stable victims reported the lowest levels of social self-competence, though by Time 3, late onset victims and desisters reported similarly low levels of social self-competence.

Stable victims initially (Time 1) reported the lowest levels of trust in their friendships. At this time, non-victims and late onset victims reported more trust in their friendships than stable victims or desisters. By Time 3, only late onset victims reported lower levels of trust in their friendships than non-victims. Late onset victims reported decreasing levels of trust from Time 1 to Time 3, $F(1, 1448) = 6.40, p < .05$.

Stable victims reported the lowest levels of affection in their relationships at Time 1. At this time, desisters reported less affection than non-victims, but similar levels of affection to late onset victims. Even before late onset victims' victimization increased, the level of affection in their friendships was similar

TABLE 3. Means (and Standard Deviations) for Friendship Variables

Time of testing	Non-victims	Desisters	Late onset victims	Stable victims
Social self-competence				
1	3.17 (0.63)[a]	2.77 (0.71)[b]	3.06 (0.81)[b]	2.17 (0.93)[c]
2	3.26 (0.62)[a]	2.94 (0.75)[b]	2.97 (0.65)[b]	2.02 (1.03)[c]
3	3.30 (0.61)[a]	3.04 (0.79)[b]	2.87 (0.74)[b]	2.78 (0.92)[b]
Trust				
1	4.15 (0.64)[a]	3.81 (0.77)[b]	4.21 (0.55)[a]	3.29 (1.45)[c]
2	4.24 (0.65)	4.18 (0.73)	4.12 (0.65)	3.66 (1.47)
3	4.19 (0.66)[a]	4.01 (0.85)	3.84 (0.88)[b]	4.00 (0.90)
Affection				
1	4.35 (0.75)[a]	3.95 (0.83)[b]	4.30 (0.67)[a]	3.44 (1.40)[c]
2	4.37 (0.71)	4.29 (0.78)	4.30 (0.72)	3.72 (1.52)
3	4.29 (0.71)[a]	4.17 (0.91)[a]	3.87 (1.01)[b]	4.17 (0.94)
Alienation				
1	2.21 (0.83)	2.40 (0.71)	2.48 (0.69)	3.03 (1.09)
2	1.97 (0.74)	1.92 (0.66)	2.13 (0.75)	2.24 (0.98)
3	1.98 (0.77)	2.05 (0.94)	2.23 (0.74)	2.53 (0.64)

Note. Means in the same row that do not share subscripts differ at $p < .05$.

to students' who were reporting high levels of victimization. By Time 3, late onset victims reported less affection than non-victims or desisters. Late onset victims reported decreasing affection over time, $F(1, 1448) = 6.17, p < .05$.

The MANCOVA analysis also revealed significant main effects of group, multivariate $F(21, 2160) = 3.07, p < .001$, with univariate effects for social self-competence, $F(3, 724) = 14.13, p < .001$; trust, $F(3, 724) = 4.26, p < .01$; alienation, $F(3, 724) = 3.77, p < .05$; and affection, $F(3, 724) = 4.33, p < .01$. Non-victims and stable victims reported the highest and lowest levels of social self-competence, respectively. Stable victims reported lower trust and affection than either non-victims or desisters. The reverse is true of alienation, for which stable victims reported higher levels.

Participants on different victimization trajectories reported differences in friendship quality with highly victimized adolescents reporting lower quality relationships than participants with low levels of victimization. As well, there is some evidence that low levels of affection in friendships are associated with subsequent increases in victimization.

Self-reported aggression and bullying. Results from the MANCOVA investigating the effects of group membership on aggression and bullying showed a significant time by group interaction, multivariate $F(12, 2865) = 4.80, p < .001$, with associated univariate effects for measures of aggression, $F(6, 1912) = 4.77, p < .001$; and bullying behavior, $F(6, 1912) = 7.64, p < .001$ (Table 4). At each time, non-victims reported the lowest levels of aggression. By Time 2, desisters reported less aggressive behaviors than did stable victims. By Time 3, desisters reported less aggression than did late onset victims. Desisters and late onset victims reported decreasing, $F(1, 1912) = 12.86, p < .001$, and increasing, $F(1, 1912) = 4.49, p < .05$, levels of aggression, respectively.

Whereas stable victims reported the most bullying behavior at Times 1 and 2, by Time 3, late onset and stable victims had comparably high levels of bullying. Similarly, desisters reported more bullying than late onset victims or non-victims at Time 1, though by Time 3, they reported less bullying than late onset or stable victims, and similar levels of bullying to non-victims. At Time 3, non-victims reported less bullying behavior than late onset or stable victims. Desisters had decreasing levels of bullying, $F(1, 1912) = 9.81, p < .001$, and late onset victims' bullying behavior increased over time, $F(1, 1912) = 23.12, p < .001$.

The MANCOVA analysis also revealed significant main effects of group, multivariate $F(6, 1912) = 13.25, p < .001$, with univariate effects for aggression, $F(3, 956) = 16.23, p < .001$; and bullying, $F(3, 956) = 22.26, p < .001$. Non-victims reported the lowest levels of aggression and bullying behavior. Stable victims reported the most bullying.

TABLE 4. Means (and Standard Deviations) for Aggression and Bullying

Time of testing	Non-victims	Desisters	Late onset victims	Stable victims
		Aggression		
1	0.34 (0.30)[a]	0.52 (0.33)[b]	0.48 (0.28)[b]	0.52 (0.27)[b]
2	0.33 (0.28)[a]	0.43 (0.28)[b]	0.52 (0.34)[b]	0.67 (0.40)[c]
3	0.32 (0.30)[a]	0.42 (0.28)[b]	0.65 (0.48)[c]	0.56 (0.42)[b,c]
		Bullying		
1	0.22 (0.46)[a]	0.68 (0.90)[b]	0.38 (0.43)[c]	1.11 (1.42)[d]
2	0.24 (0.57)[a]	0.44 (0.54)[b]	0.50 (0.62)[b]	0.86 (1.22)[c]
3	0.30 (0.62)[a]	0.32 (0.41)[a]	0.93 (1.12)[c]	1.07 (1.41)[c]

Note. Means in the same row that do not share subscripts differ at $p < .05$.

IMPLICATIONS AND INTERVENTION

The objectives of this study were to distinguish groups of children with unique profiles of victimization, to identify risk and protective factors associated with victimization, and to understand the consequences associated with stable victimization. Four groups were established: non-victims were children who reported consistently low levels of victimization; desisters were children who started with high levels of victimization which decreased over time; late onset victims reported increasing levels of victimization; and stable victims reported consistently high levels of victimization. Examining intra- and interpersonal differences across these groups will facilitate the identification of risk and protective factors associated with victimization. Finally, there was evidence to support a sequential relationship between aggression and victimization.

Risk Factors for Subsequent Victimization

The late onset victims provide the opportunity to examine factors that preceded increases in victimization, thereby delineating risk factors for victimization. Late onset victims could be distinguished from the other groups at Time 1 by high levels of internalizing problems and low levels of affection in peer relationships. Children reporting high levels of internalizing problems (e.g., anxiety, withdrawal, somatization) may elicit behaviors or initiate interactions that place them at risk for peer victimization. Rubin, Bukowski, and Parker (1998) proposed that withdrawn children follow a distinct developmental course to peer rejection (a form of peer victimization) that begins in late child-hood, when the peer group becomes aware of social withdrawal and judges it as atypical behavior. Observations of children indicate that bullying is more likely to occur when children are alone (Craig & Pepler, 1995). Anxious and withdrawn children may be hesitant to initiate social interactions and being isolated may suggest a lack of protection against bullying, and signal one's vulnerability. Bullies who harass anxious and withdrawn children may be rein-forced if victims continue to be isolated. The harassment may intensify or be-come more frequent because the bullying may exacerbate victims' anxiety, thereby rewarding bullies who can observe their powerful effect. Furthermore, if victims are not supported by others or do not defend themselves, not only may the harassment continue, but there will likely be no consequences for the bully. Thus, internalizing problems may identify those at risk for victimiza-tion, as well as contribute to maintaining the victimization and exacerbating internalizing problems.

Individuals reporting lower quality friendships also were at heightened risk for increasing victimization. Late onset victims rated affection similarly to desisters (when their victimization was high), indicating that prior to their victimization, late onset victims reported comparable levels of affection to those who were al-ready experiencing significant harassment. The lack of quality relationships or supportive peers may increase late onset victims' vulnerability to victimization (Hodges et al., 1997), demonstrating the protective function of friends.

Late onset victims reported decreasing levels of trust and affection as their victimization increased. While it is likely that they are vulnerable because they lack protection provided by friends, it also is possible that lower affec-tion in their friendships is a reflection of their victimization experiences. Ad-olescents who lack emotional support (i.e., intimacy and closeness) may lose trust in the friends they do have, who are ineffective at protecting them. Late onset victims likely did not engage in positive social interactions or experience companionship and support to help them practice social skills and develop a sense of interpersonal competence. Interestingly, despite experiencing less victimization, desisters did not report increasing levels of social competence over time. It is likely that although they were feeling less victimized by their peers, a sense of social competence would require more stable positive social interactions and experiences, that perhaps were only emerging among the desisters.

Protective Factors Against Victimization

Examining the characteristics of desisters and non-victims helps identify factors that protect children from peer victimization. Desisters were characterized by decreasing levels of internalizing problems, bullying, and aggressive behavior. Non-victims reported the lowest levels of internalizing problems, bullying, aggressive behavior, and were the most socially competent. Low levels of aggression and anxiety may be the most robust protective factors, since non-victims reported the lowest levels of these variables across time. Paralleling the results identifying low quality friendships as a risk factor, high quality friendships served a protective function. Friendships characterized by high levels of affection (representing warmth and intimacy) and trust buffered against victimization. Within these positive affective relationships a child may be more committed to a friend and therefore be inclined to intervene or protect them. Also, an intimate relationship may facilitate communication between friends and a supportive discussion can provide the opportunity to problem solve together about bullying.

Friends can help children identify strategies to deal with their harassment. Children are most likely to use the least effective methods (verbal and physical aggression) when responding to bullying and these responses are associated with more prolonged and severe bullying interactions (Mahady-Wilton, Craig, & Pepler, 2000). In contrast, when children ask a peer for help with the bullying, it stops within 10 seconds half the time (O'Connell, Pepler, & Craig, 1999). Because desisters report decreasing aggression over time, it is possible that they are coping in more effective ways (i.e., utilizing their friends or not responding aggressively) and these behaviors played a role in reducing victimization. The increase in aggression over time reported by late onset victims further supports this interpretation. Interventions designed to reduce aggressive behavior and offer alternate coping strategies may prevent victimization, and the negative outcomes associated with it.

Stable Victimization Associated with Aversive Conditions

Stable victims reported the most severe intra- and interpersonal difficulties. High levels of anxiety, withdrawal, somatization, bullying, and low social competence characterize this group, suggesting that long-term exposure and cumulative effects of victimization place them at increased risk for long-term problems. Without intervention the cycle of victimization will intensify. Because stable victimization is associated with the most negative conditions, treatment aimed at decreasing risk or reducing victimization should occur early.

Relationship Between Aggression and Victimization

There was a sequential relationship between aggression and victimization. As victimization increased, late onset victims reported engaging in more aggressive and bullying behaviors. Children who are targets of victimization for prolonged periods may learn and model aggressive strategies from the bullies, whom they view as more powerful. Furthermore, they may aggress against those weaker than themselves as a way of coping with their anger and hostility associated with their own victimization experiences. Responding to bullying with aggression is not an effective strategy (Mahady-Wilton et al., 2000), even though it is the most frequent response. Interventions for victimized children should provide effective coping strategies

Limitations

While the results of this study provide direction and implications for intervention, there are some limitations. Group membership and the dependent measures were both based on self-report, thus the results may be biased due to shared method variance. Previous research, however, indicates that self-reports are valid assessments of victimization (Farrington, 1993), particularly since adults and teachers tend to underestimate the problem. While results highlight the role of peer socialization in the development and maintenance of victimization, previous research acknowledges the importance of the family. This study did not evaluate parent-child relationships. Finally, participants came from highly educated, two-parent families; therefore, generalizations to other populations should be made with caution.

Implications for Research and Practice in Applied School Psychology

This study has implications for the prevention and intervention of peer victimization with respect to assessment and identification as well as specific program components. Since internalizing problems preceded victimization, children at risk for victimization can be identified with a screening tool that would assess levels of anxiety, withdrawal, and somatization, as well as victimization. Because of the cumulative effects of victimization, assessment and screening should occur early (i.e., in kindergarten) and at regular intervals. Once at-risk children are identified, school personnel and parents can intervene with individuals or peer group to decrease the risk factors and increase protective factors associated with victimization.

Targeted interventions for individual children should focus on reducing their internalizing problems, promoting interpersonal competence skills to enhance friendship initiation and maintenance, and reducing isolation and withdrawal (i.e., relaxation training, cognitive restructuring techniques to deal with anxiety provoking situations, social skills and assertiveness training). Victimized children also need to develop skills to communicate their distress in a way that promotes a positive response from peers and teachers. Teaching children specific strategies that are empirically demonstrated to be effective in stopping bullying, such as asking for help and positive conflict resolution, will reduce their risk for future victimization (O'Connell et al., 1999). Finally, education regarding the ineffectiveness of strategies such as aggression also is important.

In addition to working with individuals, programs should be directed at the peer group to encourage inclusion and foster supportive social networks. An example of a school-wide program for peers is 'support circles' which offer children the opportunity to enhance their social competence through peer interaction and support. Small groups of students discuss regularly everyday events or personal concerns and problems. These opportunities help children to develop intimate and affectionate relationships that promote support and protection and may prevent future victimization. Through the creation of these groups, at-risk children and victimized children will have regular opportunities to interact with skilled peers, practice and develop their social skills, develop social competence, and acquire the peer support and protection they may lack. Another example of this type of intervention is mentoring programs whereby small groups of students meet with a teacher to address nonacademic concerns in a safe and non-judgmental environment, creating a supportive context to discuss interpersonal matters. Finally, classroom discussions can identify prosocial strategies for intervening in bullying and emphasize the critical role and responsibility of the peer group in stopping the harassment by supporting and standing up for the victims. When bullying problems occur, teachers can focus on the nature of the peer involvement and identify the role that peers may play in exacerbating the problem. By encouraging the entire peer group to take responsibility for harassment, it should encourage individuals to intervene on behalf of victims.

In summary, the implications of this research are: (1) victims should be identified early though regular screenings that assess internalizing problems and friendship quality; (2) interventions to reduce victimization should include specific elements that address intra- and interpersonal risk and protective factors (i.e., be systemic and include individuals as well as the peer group).

REFERENCES

Achenbach, T. M. (1991). *Manual for the Youth Self-Report and 1991 Profile.* Burlington, VT: University of Vermont Department of Psychiatry.

Armsden, G. C., & Greenberg, M. T. (1987). The inventory of parent and peer attachment: Individual differences and their relationship to psychological well-being in adolescence. *Journal of Youth and Adolescence, 16,* 427-454.

Austin, S., & Joseph, S. (1996). Assessment of bully/victim problems in 8- to 11-year-olds. *British Journal of Educational Psychology, 66*(4), 447-456.

Boulton, M. J., & Underwood, K. (1992). Bully/victim problems among middle school children. *British Journal of Educational Psychology, 62*, 73-87.

Charach, A., Pepler, D., & Ziegler, S. (1995). Bullying at school: A Canadian perspective. *Education Canada, 35*(1), 12-18.

Craig, W. M. (1998). The relationship among bullying, victimization, depression, anxiety, and aggression in elementary school children. *Journal of Personality and Individual Differences, 24*(1), 123-130.

Craig, W. M., & Pepler, D. J. (1995). Peer processes in bullying and victimization: An observational study. *Exceptionality Education in Canada, 5*, 81-95.

Farrington, D. P. (1993). Understanding and preventing bullying. In Tonry, M. & Morris, N. (Eds.), *Crime and Justice, 17*, 381-458. Chicago: University of Chicago Press.

Furman, W., & Buhrmester, D. (1985). Children's perceptions of the personal relationships in their social networks. *Developmental Psychology, 21*, 1016-1024.

Goldbaum, S., & Craig, W. M. (2001, April). *Analyzing Trajectories of Victimization: A Developmental Perspective.* Poster session presented at the Society for Research on Child Development, Minneapolis, MN.

Harter, S. (1982). The Perceived Competence Scale for Children. *Child Development, 53*, 87-97.

Hartup, W. W. (1992). Peer relations in early and middle childhood. In V. B. Van Hasselt & M. Herson (Eds.), *Handbook of Social Development: A Lifespan Perspective* (pp. 257-281). New York: Plenum.

Hodges, E. V., Boivin, M., Vitaro, F., & Bukowski, W. (1999). The power of friendship: Protection against an escalating cycle of peer victimization. *Developmental Psychology, 35*(1), 94-101.

Hodges, E. V., Malone, M. J., & Perry, D. G. (1997). Individual risk and social risk as interacting determinants of victimization in the peer group. *Developmental Psychopathology, 33*(6), 1032-1039.

Kochenderfer, B. J., & Ladd, G. W. (1997). Victimized children's responses to peers' aggression: Behaviors associated with reduced versus continued victimization. *Development and Psychopathology, 9*, 59-73.

Kumpulainen, K., Raesaenen, E., & Henttonen, I. (1999). Children involved in bullying: Psychological disturbance and the persistence of the involvement. *Child Abuse and Neglect, 23*(12), 1253-1262.

Mahady Wilton, M. M., Craig, W. M., & Pepler, D. J. (2000). Emotional regulations and display in classroom victims of bullying: Characteristic expressions of affect, coping styles and relevant contextual factors. *Social Development, 9*(2), 226-244.

Nagin, D. (1999). Analyzing developmental trajectories: A semiparametric group-based approach. *Psychological Methods, 4*(2), 139-157.

Nagin, D., & Tremblay, R. E. (1999). Trajectories of boys' physical aggression, opposition, and hyperactivity on the path to physically violent and nonviolent juvenile delinquency. *Child Development, 70*(5), 1181-1196.

O'Connell, P., Pepler, D. J., & Craig, W. M. (1999). Peer involvement in bullying: Insights and challenges for intervention. *Journal of Adolescence, 22*(4), 437-452.

Olweus, D. (1991). Bully/victim problems among schoolchildren: Basic facts and effects of a school based intervention program. In Debra J. Pepler & Kenneth H. Rubin (Eds.), *The Development and Treatment of Childhood Aggression* (pp. 411-448). NJ: Lawrence Erlbaum Associates, Inc.

Olweus, D. (1993). Victimization by peers: Antecedents and long-term outcomes. In K. H. Rubin & J. B. Asendorpf (Eds.), *Social Withdrawal, Inhibition, and Shyness in Childhood* (pp. 315-341). Hillsdale, NJ: Erlbaum.

Parker, J. G., & Asher, S. R. (1987). Peer relations and later personal adjustment: Are low-accepted children at risk? *Psychological Bulletin, 102*(3), 357-389.

Pellegrini, A. D. (1998). Bullies and victims in school: A review and call for research. *Journal of Applied Developmental Psychology, 19*(2), 165-176.

Rubin, K. H., Bukowski, W., & Parker, J. G. (1998). In W. Damon & N. Eisenberg (Eds.), *Handbook of Child Psychology, 5th Edition: Social, Emotional, and Personality Development* (pp. 619-699). New York: John Wiley & Sons.

Salmivalli, C., Huttunen, A., & Lagerspetz, M. J. (1997). Peer networks and bullying in schools. *Scandinavian Journal of Psychology, 38*, 305-312.

Straus, M. A. (1979). Measuring intrafamily conflict and violence: The Conflict Tactics Scale. *Journal of Marriage and the Family, 41*, 75-88.

Bullying Is Power:
Implications for School-Based
Intervention Strategies

Tracy Vaillancourt

McMaster University

Shelley Hymel

University of British Columbia

Patricia McDougall

University of Saskatchewan

SUMMARY. The present investigation examines subtypes of bullies, distinguished on the basis of social power, some of whom fit the tradi-

Address correspondence to: Tracy Vaillancourt, PhD, Department of Psychology, McMaster University, 1280 Main Street West, Hamilton, Ontario, Canada (E-mail: vaillat@mcmaster.ca).

The research reported herein was collected as part of the doctoral dissertation of the first author and with support provided through the University of British Columbia Hampton Research Fund. Portions of this research were presented at the first annual British Columbia Ministry of Education Research Symposium, Vancouver, Canada, in February of 2001 (Vaillancourt & Hymel, 2001) and at the XVth World Meeting for the Society for Research on Aggression, Montreal, Canada, in July 2002 (Vaillancourt, Rodkin, Hymel, McDougall, Bonnano, & Welch, 2002).

The authors wish to thank the students who participated in this research, and the administrators, teachers, staff and parents who enthusiastically supported this project, with particular recognition of Vice Principal Richard Bahan's efforts to make the project a reality.

[Haworth co-indexing entry note]: "Bullying Is Power: Implications for School-Based Intervention Strategies." Vaillancourt, Tracy, Shelley Hymel, and Patricia McDougall. Co-published simultaneously in *Journal of Applied School Psychology* (The Haworth Press, Inc.) Vol. 19, No. 2, 2003, pp. 157-176; and: *Bullying, Peer Harassment, and Victimization in the Schools: The Next Generation of Prevention* (ed: Maurice J. Elias, and Joseph E. Zins) The Haworth Press, Inc., 2003, pp. 157-176. Single or multiple copies of this article are available for a fee from The Haworth Document Delivery Service [1-800-HAWORTH, 9:00 a.m. - 5:00 p.m. (EST). E-mail address: docdelivery@haworthpress.com].

10.1300/J008v19n02_10

tional characterization of bullies as poorly accepted, psychologically troubled, marginal members of the peer group and others who exhibit a much more positive set of social characteristics and who are afforded high status within the peer group. In a sample of 555 grade 6 to 10 Canadian students, the associations between bullying, power, and social status were examined, as well as variability in bullies across behavioral and non-behavioral characteristics, self-perceptions, and mental health functioning. Peer nominations were used to assess bullying, social status, aggressive behavior, competencies and assets, and self-reports were used to assess social self-perceptions and internalizing difficulties. Results indicated that, although generally viewed by peers as disliked and aggressive, a substantial number of bullies were also seen as both popular and powerful with leadership qualities, competencies and assets. In terms of their own social self-perceptions, bullies reported feeling good about themselves and their peer interactions. When subgroups of bullies were distinguished in terms of varying levels of perceived social power, powerful bullies were perceived by peers to be more popular, better liked and more physically and relationally aggressive than low power bullies. Additionally, powerful bullies were viewed as exhibiting more competencies and assets such as being physically attractive, wearing stylish clothing, and being good athletes. Findings are discussed in terms of the perpetuation of bullying behavior and the implications of the present findings for anti-bullying interventions. *[Article copies available for a fee from The Haworth Document Delivery Service: 1-800-HAWORTH. E-mail address: <docdelivery@haworthpress.com> Website: <http://www.HaworthPress.com> © 2003 by The Haworth Press, Inc. All rights reserved.]*

KEYWORDS. Bullying, popularity, peer relations, harassment, social status

Much of what is known about bullies and bullying behavior comes from Olweus' (1973, 1978, 1993, 1996) large scale studies of Scandinavian children in which he distinguished bullies from non-involved students or victims in terms of their positive views of violence and of themselves (high rather than low self-esteem), their impulsivity and physical strength, and their lack of insecurity, anxiety and empathy for victims. More recent studies have focused on the mental health functioning of children identified as bullies. Like victims, bullies are at risk for internalizing difficulties including depression, suicidal ideation (e.g., Kaltiala-Heino, Rimpela, Marttunen, Rimpela, & Rantanen,

1999), and loneliness (e.g., Forero & McLellan, 1999), and like aggressive children, bullies are at risk for externalizing disorders (e.g., Kumpulainen et al., 1998), delinquency and criminality (e.g., Olweus, 1993), as well as poor academic achievement, smoking, and substance abuse (e.g., Nansel et al., 2001). These findings are consistent with traditional, intuitive notions of bullies as poorly accepted, marginal members of the peer group who are psychologically unfit. We question this stereotypic portrayal of bullies, and suggest that there are distinct subtypes of bullies, differentiated in terms of their social power and status.

Issues of social power are critical to understanding the complex nature of bullying. Despite the fact that current definitions of bullying emphasize the power differential that exists within bully-victim relationships as a key characteristic of bullying (e.g., Besag, 1989; Olweus, 1993, 1996), there has been little, if any, systematic investigation of the links between bullying and power, and little appreciation of the fact that social power reflects an interaction between the characteristics of the individual and the social context in which he/she operates. Accordingly, the present study distinguishes different subtypes of bullies on the basis of their perceived power within the group. Our hypotheses regarding bullying subtypes are based on a distinction between implicit and explicit social power made by LaFreniere and Charlesworth (1983). Explicit social power "is expressed explicitly and forcefully and thereby elicits fear, submission, or compliance"; implicit social power "stems from a recognition of status or competence and thereby depends upon acceptance by subordinates" (p. 66). We believe that all bullies rely on explicit social power to some degree, using such things as greater size and strength and various forms of aggressive behaviour to coerce peers who, in turn, are submissive as a result of fear. However, some bullies also possess characteristics and assets that are valued by the peer group and, as a result, these bullies are afforded a high degree of status within the group, giving them implicit social power. In both cases, bullies may be granted a certain degree of dominance and influence within the peer group, but for different reasons. Moreover, relative reliance on implicit versus explicit social power may contribute to social status within the peer group, with implicit social power associated with greater status.

Critical to understanding the relationship between bullying and status is the distinction made by Parkhurst and Hopmeyer (1998) between sociometric acceptance/rejection (operationalized as the degree to which one is generally liked versus disliked by peers) and peer perceptions of "popularity" or status within the group. In their study of early adolescents, Parkhurst and Hopmeyer found that these two status indicators, both derived from peer assessments, were significantly but modestly related ($r = .28$), with only 36% of sociometrically accepted or well-liked students actually being perceived as "popular." Moreover, some disliked or rejected students (11%) and nearly half of the "controversial" students (liked by some, disliked by others) were perceived as "popular." Thus, sociometric liking/disliking is not necessarily synonymous with perceived status or popularity; being rejected is not the same as being viewed by peers as unpopular or low in status.

With regard to the social status of bullies, early studies by Olweus (1973, 1978, 1993) found bullies to be average in terms of peer liking, although this "acceptance" was rather short lived, as the majority of bullies were disliked by their peers once they reached the later elementary and high school years. Other studies generally have found bullies to be disliked or rejected by their peers (Boulton, 1999; Boulton & Smith, 1994; Pelligrini, Bartini, & Brooks, 1999). Similar associations have been documented between aggression and peer rejection (see Rubin, Bukowski, & Parker, 1998), although the magnitude of this relationship is modest, with only about 50% of aggressive children actually being rejected by peers (e.g., Rubin et al., 1998). At least some aggressive children and adolescents are actually solid and central members of their social clique (e.g., Farmer & Rodkin, 1996), are liked by their peers (e.g., Hess & Aiken, 1998), and are perceived as popular or highly visible and prominent within the peer group (e.g., Estell, Cairns, Farmer, & Cairns, 2002; Vaillancourt & Hymel, 2002). Recent ethnographic studies (e.g., Adler & Adler, 1998; Merten, 1997) also demonstrate links between cruel and aggressive behavior and high levels of status and popularity within the peer group.

In light of this research, we hypothesized that, like aggressive children and adolescents, bullies are generally disliked by their peers, owing primarily to the fact that all bullies rely to some degree on explicit social power (i.e., aggression). However, some bullies are also perceived as popular and powerful as a function of their access to implicit social power. Following from the argument that possession of peer-valued characteristics provides the basis for implicit social power, we hypothesized that bullies who wield implicit social power would differ from those who do not in terms of their level of perceived social status and their possession of certain competencies and assets that are valued by the peer group. Of additional interest was whether subtypes of bullies would also differ in terms of their own social self-perceptions and indices of mental well-being, with more favorable perceptions and outcomes expected for those bullies who enjoy high levels of power. Understanding these relationships between power, status and bullying is critical to informing intervention efforts aimed at reducing bullying in schools.

METHOD

Participants

As part of a larger longitudinal project, students in grades 6 to 10 (age range = 11-17 years) were recruited from all five elementary schools (grades K-7) and the only secondary school (grades 8-12) that serviced a moderate-sized, western Canadian city (population approx. 9,000). All participants received parental consent (270 girls, 285 boys; M age = 13.3 years, SD = 1.49 years), with approximately equal numbers across grades and an overall participation rate of 95%. The sample was predominantly White (93%), with a small percentage of First Nations, Asian Canadian, Indo Canadian, and Latin Canadian students, reflecting the makeup of the community.

Procedures

Students participated in a single group-testing session (50 minutes) during which they completed both self-report and peer assessment measures, as described below. Participants were assured of the confidentiality of their individual responses to all measures.

Peer Assessment Measures

Students were asked to nominate an unlimited[1] number of grade-mates of either sex who best fit each of 40 sociometric, behavioral, and non-behavioral descriptors, as described in Table 1. For each item, nominations received from grade-mates were summed and standardized within grade to yield a continuous measure of the characteristic assessed. In some cases (see Table 1), conceptually related items were averaged to create composite indices, computed as the sum of standardized items divided by the number of items in the composite. For each construct, higher scores reflected greater peer perceptions of the characteristic described.

Peer nominations were used to assess perceptions of bullying behavior, with higher scores indicating that a greater number of peers viewed that person as a bully. Although self-report data are often used to identify bullies (e.g., Olweus, 1994; Rigby, 1999), peer nominations represent a more time-consuming, but face valid alternative (e.g., Perry, Kusel, & Perry, 1988) that avoids potential self-reporting biases (e.g., denial, exaggeration) and reflects the perspective of multiple informants within students' primary social context. Peer nominations were also used to assess perceived power using a composite of two items, and to assess three different indices of social status: perceived pop-

TABLE 1. Peer Assessment Measure

Construct	Item(s)	Internal Consistency	Range of Scores (unstandardized proportion scores)[1]
Bullying	Who is a bully?		0-91% of peers
Power	Who seems to have a lot of power over others? +Who can pressure others into doing things?	alpha = .83	0-83% of peers
Social Status Perceived Popularity	Who are the most popular people in your grade?		0-96% of peers
Liking/Acceptance	Who are the people you like most in your grade?		0-63% of peers
Disliking/Rejection	Who are the people you like least in your grade?		0-65% of peers
Aggressive Behavior Physical Aggression	Who starts fights and arguments with others? +Who hits, pushes others?	alpha = .86	0-76% of peers
Relational Aggression	Who spreads rumors about someone to get others to stop liking the person? +Who tries to control or dominate a person by excluding them from the peer group? +Who tells others to stop liking a person to get even with them? +Who ignores people when they are mad at them (gives people the silent treatment)? +Who will make someone feel bad or look bad by making a face, turning away, or rolling their eyes?	alpha = .86	0-35% of peers
Competencies and Assets Prosocial Behavior	Who always gets along well with other people? +Who is able to understand other people's point of view? +Who is helpful and cooperative? +Who is kind and nice to others? +Who helps others when they have a problem?	alpha = .89	0-38% of peers
Leadership	Who is a good leader?		0-70% of peers
Wealth	Who seems to be rich?		0-92% of peers
Appearance	Who is good looking or attractive? +Who dresses well and is in style?	alpha = .86	0-63% of peers
Athletic competence	Who does well in sports?		0-88% of peers
Academic competence	Who does well in their schoolwork?		0-91% of peers

[1] Unstandardized proportion scores reflect the extent to which individuals were perceived by their peers to possess the behavioral or non-behavioral characteristics in question. For example, the range of scores of 0-91% obtained for the bullying item indicates that at least one participant was nominated as a bully by 91% of her/his grade-mates.

ularity (succeeding Parkhurst & Hopmeyer, 1998) and the more traditional sociometric indices of peer liking (acceptance) and disliking (rejection). Following previous research (Coie & Dodge, 1983; Crick & Grotpeter, 1995; Galen & Underwood, 1997), peer nomination composites were also used to assess both physical aggression (i.e., hitting), and relational aggression, defined as social manipulation that is intended to harm (i.e., spreading rumors; Crick & Grotpeter, 1995). Finally, peer nomination data were used to assess six assets or competencies: prosocial behavior, leadership, appearance, wealth, academic and athletic competence, with higher scores reflecting peer perceptions of greater levels of competence or assets in each case.

Self-Report Measures

Self-report questionnaires were used to assess both social self-perceptions and internalizing difficulties. Specifically, social self-efficacy, or the degree to which a person believes he/she can evoke change within a social context, was measured using a 5-item scale adapted for adolescents (Sletta, 1998) from Wheeler and Ladd's (1982) *Social Self-Efficacy Scale* ($\alpha = .74$; $M = 17.67$, $SD = 3.85$). Perceptions of peer social support were assessed using two 7-item subscales of the *Relational Provisions Loneliness Questionnaire* developed by Hayden (1989, see Terrell-Deutsch, 1999), one assessing perceived intimacy (having others to confide in; $\alpha = .85$; $M = 28.92$, $SD = 5.93$) and one assessing perceived integration or belonging (having others to hang out and do things with; $\alpha = .89$; $M = 28.62$, $SD = 5.57$). The 8-item social self-concept subscale of the *Self-Description Questionnaire I (SDQI*; Marsh, 1988) was used to assess the extent to which students held positive opinions of their peer interactions (e.g., "Most other kids like me"; $\alpha = .90$; $M = 31.18$, $SD = 6.40$). Depression was assessed using a 26-item adaptation (one item on suicide deleted at the request of the schools) of the *Child Depression Inventory* (Kovacs, 1991/92; $\alpha = .89$; $M = 35.74$, $SD = 8.58$), while students' feelings of loneliness were assessed using the 16-item, *Loneliness and Social Dissatisfaction Scale* (Asher, Hymel, & Renshaw, 1984; $\alpha = .88$; $M = 28.41$, $SD = 9.67$). Finally, the extent to which students held global, positive perceptions of self was assessed using the general self-worth subscale of the *SDQ I* ($\alpha = .86$; $M = 33.28$, $SD = 5.15$).

RESULTS

Characteristics Associated with Bullying and Power

Zero-order correlational analyses were first conducted to examine the relationships among bullying, power, and various indices of *status* (popularity, liking, disliking), *aggressive behavior* (relational, physical), *competencies and assets* (appearance, wealth, athletic and academic competence, prosocial behavior, leadership), *social self-perceptions* (social self-efficacy, peer intimacy, peer integration, social self-concept) and *internalizing difficulties* (depression, loneliness, general self-worth) across the entire sample. Results indicated that peer perceptions of bullying were significantly related to a broad range of peer-assessed characteristics (degrees of freedom range from 524-553; all p's $< .001$ unless otherwise indicated), although the magnitude of these correlations varied considerably. As expected, children identified as bullies were generally viewed by peers as more powerful ($r = .67$) and, to a lesser extent, as more popular ($r = .29$), although they were also generally disliked ($r = .32$). Not surprisingly, bullies were viewed by peers as more physically ($r = .79$) and relationally aggressive ($r = .50$). With regard to positive competencies and assets, bullying was significantly, but only minimally associated with peer perceptions of greater leadership ($r = .21$), athletic competence ($r = .14$) and appearance ($r = .18$), as well as less prosocial behavior ($r = -.17$) and lower academic competence ($r = -.12$; p = .006$). The low magnitude of these correlations suggests that each of these positive characteristics is not evident across all students identified as bullies. With regard to self-perceptions and internalizing difficulties, peer-identified bullies reported feeling more socially competent ($r = .13$, $p = .004$) and efficacious ($r = .23$). Bullying was not significantly related to depression ($r = .06$), general self-worth ($r = .05$) loneliness ($r = -.08$), liking ($r = .03$), wealth ($r = .04$), or perceptions of peer social support in the form of intimacy ($r = .03$) or integration ($r = .08$).

A similar pattern of correlations was observed when peer ratings of power were considered. On the positive side, greater power was associated with being popular ($r = .58$), frequently liked ($r = .22$), and less disliked by peers ($r = -.19$). Similarly, perceived power was associated with better appearance ($r = .46$), wealth ($r = .19$), athleticism ($r = .27$), and leadership (r = .42). Higher power, however, was also linked to more aggressive behavior in both physical ($r = .57$) and relational forms ($r = .57$). Like the self-perceptions of bullies, students with higher power reported greater social self-efficacy ($r = .26$) and competence with peers ($r = .22$). But unlike bullies, students viewed by peers as powerful saw themselves as better integrated within the peer group ($r = .16$), less lonely ($r = -.17$) and were higher in general self-worth ($r = .14$). Power was not significantly related to peer nominations of academic competence ($r = -.07$), prosocial behavior ($r = -.04$), perceptions of peer intimacy ($r = .08$) or reports of depression ($r = .02$).

Given our interest in demonstrating a link between bullying and power, we wanted to ensure that power was not synonymous with other peer nominated characteristics or behaviors (e.g., aggression). Specifically, we sought to examine whether power would continue to be predictive of bullying even when the effects of other related peer nominations were partialled out. In a simultaneous regression analysis with indices of peer status, aggressive behavior and competencies as predictors, we were able to account for 69% of the variability in peer nominations of bullying ($F(12, 522) = 96.76, p < .001$). After controlling for the effects of other peer nominations, power ($p = .297$; semi-partial (sr) = .18, $p < .001$), relational aggression ($p = .089$; $sr = .07, p = .008$), physical aggression ($p = .579$; $sr = .43, p < .001$), and leadership ($p = .066$, $sr = .05, p = .042$) remained uniquely predictive (all p's < .001) of bullying. Thus, despite the fact that both leadership and aggressive behavior appear to be important correlates of bullying, power makes a unique contribution and is not simply redundant with aggression and leadership qualities.

Creating Subtypes of Bullies

Of primary interest here was consideration of the characteristics associated with bullying. To this end, a sub-sample of students identified as bullies by their peers was selected, operationally defined as those who scored at or above 1/2 standard deviation of the mean for their grade on the item, "Who is a bully?" Our use of the 1/2 standard deviation as a cutoff criterion follows from the work of Schwartz (2000). Of these bullies, 44 were in elementary school, 58 were in secondary school, and 33 were girls, 69 were boys.

Subsequent analyses examined whether the characteristics associated with bullying varied as a function of sex (girls vs. boys) and school context (elementary vs. secondary school). Specifically, for the sub-sample of 102 peer-identified bullies, a series of 2 (sex) × 2 (school context) MANOVAs were conducted using the following dependent variables: (1) peer nominations of bullying, (2) aggressive behaviors (intercorrelation $r = .48$), (3) social status (intercorrelations among variables ranged from −.01 to .44), (4) competencies and assets (intercorrelations ranged from .06 to .46), (5) social self-perceptions (intercorrelations ranged from .27 to .80) and (6) internalizing difficulties (intercorrelations ranged from .35 to −.46).

Results of these analyses revealed one significant multivariate interaction between sex and school context for *aggressive behaviors* (Wilks's = .88, $F(2,91) = 6.07, p = .003, \eta^2 = 12$) and one significant main effect at the multivariate level, also for *aggressive behaviors* (Wilks's = .88, $F(2,91) = 5.95, p = .004, \eta^2 = 12$), along with significant main effects of sex in the domains of *aggressive behaviors* (Wilks's $\lambda = .66, F(2, 91) = 23.29, p < .001, \eta^2 = .34$), *competencies and assets* (Wilks's $\lambda = .73, F(6, 88) = 5.35, p < .01, \eta^2 = .27$), and *social self-perceptions* (Wilks's $\lambda = .84, F(4, 85) = 3.94, p = .006, \eta^2 = $

.16). Follow-up ANOVAs indicated that the sex by school context interaction was significant for *physical aggression* $(F(1,92) = 6.03, p = .016, \eta^2 = .06)$. Although peer reports of physical aggression declined from elementary to secondary school for boys $(M = 1.80, SD = 1.15; M = .76, SD = 1.25,$ respectively), this shift was not significant for girls $(M = .57, SD = .72$ elementary; $M = 1.10, SD = 1.38$ secondary). In contrast, the main effect of context for *relational aggression* $(F(1,92) = 11.82, p = .001, \eta^2 = .11)$ revealed a decrease in the use this type of aggression for both girls and boys from elementary $(M = .85, SD = .90)$ to high school $(M = .37, SD = .63)$. Finally, follow-up ANOVAs showed sex differences for relational aggression $(F(1,96) = 24.89, p < .001, \eta^2 = .21)$, *athletic competence* $(F(1,93) = 5.35, p = .023, \eta^2 = .05)$, *appearance* $(F(1,93) = 4.92, p = .029, \eta2 = .05)$ and *peer intimacy* $(F(1, 88) = 10.71, p = .002, \eta2 = .11)$. Female bullies were seen as more relationally aggressive $(M = 5.44, SD = 4.52)$, yet reported higher peer intimacy $(M = 31.81, SD = 5.49)$ as compared to male bullies $(M = 1.78, SD = 3.00,$ and $M = 27.74, SD = 5.68;$ respectively). Further, male bullies were viewed as more athletic $(M = .23, SD = 1.01)$ but less attractive $(M = .15, SD = 1.94)$ than female bullies $(M = -.15, SD = .67$ and $M = 1.16, SD = 2.2;$ respectively).

Differences in Power: Subtypes of Bullies

As mentioned previously, our central interest was in the identification of subtypes of bullies who were expected to vary in terms of a number of characteristics. Accordingly, the 102 peer-identified bullies were classified into one of three subgroups, based on peer reports of power. Bullies who scored at or above standard deviation of the mean for their grade on perceived power were categorized as highly powerful, whereas bullies who scored at or below 1/2 standard deviation of the mean were categorized as having low power. Bullies with perceived power scores within ± 1/2 standard deviation of the mean were categorized as moderate in power. Using these criteria, we identified 10 low power bullies (1 girl, 9 boys), 41 moderately powerful bullies (15 girls, 26 boys), and 51 highly powerful bullies (17 girls, 34 boys). Of interest was whether these subgroups differed in terms of behavioral and non-behavioral characteristics.

Subgroup differences for both relational and physical aggression were assessed using a one-way MANOVA. Results (see Table 2) revealed significant differences in *aggressive behavior* (Wilks's $\lambda = .84, F(4, 182) = 4.33, p = .002, \eta^2 = .09$), with follow-up univariate ANOVAs and post-hoc LSD tests showing that highly powerful bullies were viewed as more relationally aggressive $(F(2, 93) = 7.70, p = .001, \eta^2 = .14)$ as compared to moderate and low power bullies. Powerful bullies also demonstrated a tendency toward being seen as

TABLE 2. Differences Across Bullying Subgroups (Unadjusted Means)

	High Power Bully ($n = 51$) [1]average proportion = 16%		Moderate Power Bully ($n = 41$) average proportion = 3%		Low Power Bully ($n = 10$) average proportion = 0%		
	M	(SD)	M	(SD)	M	(SD)	[2]Post-hoc Comparisons
Aggressive Behavior	1.27	(1.24)	0.94	(1.20)	0.34	(0.88)	Trend HI > LO
Physical Aggression	0.87	(0.82)	0.42	(0.72)	0.04	(0.34)	HI > MOD, LO
Relational Aggression							
Social Status	1.32	(1.58)	−0.16	(0.58)	−0.29	(0.29)	HI > MOD, LO
Perceived Popularity	0.40	(1.03)	−0.29	(0.81)	−0.08	(1.14)	HI > MOD
Liked Most	0.46	(.79)	0.51	(1.18)	0.18	(0.92)	
Liked Least							
Competencies and Assets	0.69	(1.32)	−0.17	(0.48)	−0.32	(0.17)	HI > MOD, LO
Appearance	0.18	(1.13)	−0.10	(0.72)	0.07	(0.55)	
Wealth	0.33	(1.11)	0.01	(0.80)	−0.43	(0.06)	
Athleticism	−0.22	(0.41)	−0.42	(0.37)	−0.20	(0.57)	
Prosocial Behavior	0.93	(1.52)	−0.28	(0.47)	−0.47	(0.47)	HI > MOD, LO
Leadership	−0.25	(0.57)	−0.35	(0.22)	−0.26	(0.42)	
Academic							
Social Self-Perceptions	20.00	(3.08)	18.89	(4.41)	18.11	(3.92)	
Self-Efficacy	29.42	(5.84)	29.23	(5.48)	24.78	(7.16)	
Intimacy	28.93	(7.03)	28.69	(5.28)	26.44	(5.10)	
Integration	33.67	(6.42)	31.14	(7.40)	28.44	(2.79)	
Peer Self-Concept							
Internalizing Difficulties	38.79	(8.79)	37.69	(10.69)	36.44	(8.47)	
Depression	26.23	(8.91)	29.75	(10.42)	30.67	(14.20)	
Loneliness	33.36	(6.18)	33.44	(5.51)	30.11	(4.11)	
General Self-Worth							

Note. 1. Average proportion scores represent the percentage of students in the nominating network who perceived the individual as powerful. For example, students in the moderate power group were, on average, viewed as powerful by 5% of their peer network. 2. HI = High power, MOD = Moderate power, LO = Low power bully.

more physically aggressive ($F(2, 93) = 2.73, p = .071, \eta^2 = .06$) as compared to bullies with low power.

Given the strong zero-order associations observed between bullying, power and aggressive behavior and the fact that relational and physical aggression emerged as uniquely predictive of bullying in our regression analysis, efforts to control for aggressive behavior were undertaken in subsequent analyses examining variations across bullying subgroups. Our goal was to examine characteristics of various subtypes of bullies that reflect variations in implicit power, not explicit power exerted through aggressive behavior. A series of one-way MANCOVAs were conducted examining differences across the three bullying subgroups in terms of (1) social status, (2) competencies and assets, (3) social self-perceptions, and (4) self-reported internalizing difficulties, after covarying out the effects of relational and physical aggression. Results (see Table 2) indicated significant differences in *social status*, Wilks's $\lambda = .71$, $F(6, 176) = 5.39$, $p < .001$, $\eta^2 = .16$, and *competencies and assets*, Wilks's $\lambda = .74$, $F(12, 162) = 2.16$, $p = .016$, $\eta^2 = .14$. No statistically significant differences were observed across subtypes for social self-perceptions or internalizing difficulties.

Follow-up univariate tests for *social status* revealed that variations in peer liking and perceived popularity were both statistically significant ($F(2, 90) = 5.53$, $p = .005$, $\eta^2 = .11$ and $F(2, 90) = 16.82$, $p < .001$, $\eta^2 = .27$; respectively), with LSD post-hoc tests on adjusted means indicating that powerful bullies were perceived as more popular than moderate or low power bullies. Similarly, bullies with high power were better liked than moderate power bullies. For *competencies and assets*, follow-up ANCOVAs revealed significant variations across bullying subtypes for leadership ($F(2, 86) = 11.84$, $p < .001$, $\eta^2 = .22$) and appearance ($F(2, 86) = 6.56$, $p = .002$, $\eta^2 = .13$). Results of LSD post-hoc tests on adjusted means showed that powerful bullies were viewed more favorably by their peers, who saw them as more attractive (e.g., stylish) and as better leaders compared to moderate and low power bullies.

DISCUSSION

Definitions of bullying emphasize the power differential that exists between bullies and their victims. In the present study, we verify the link between bullying and perceived power within the adolescent peer group. Although not synonymous, bullying and power are linked in significant and complex ways. In the present sample, many (if not most) of the bullies identified by peers did not fit the stereotype of a psychologically maladjusted, marginalized individual. Rather, correlational results indicated that bullies in this study were considered both popular and powerful, even if they were generally disliked. Given their apparent high status within the peer group, it is not surprising that, overall, bullies reported a positive sense of social self-efficacy, and a positive social self-concept. Further, peer nominated bullies also reported feeling well integrated with the peer group and less lonely. Consistent with Olweus (1993, 1996), peer identified bullies in this study did not report lower self-esteem. However, in contrast to previous research suggesting that bullies may be at risk for depression (e.g., Roland, 2002), peer-identified bullies in this study did not report greater levels of depression.

When the sex of the bully was considered, an interesting yet predictable pattern of results emerged. Specifically, consistent with what has been found with aggressive children (e.g., Crick & Grotpeter, 1995), female bullies in the present study were viewed by peers as being more relationally aggressive and less physically aggressive than male bullies. Moreover, female bullies reported greater peer intimacy than male bullies, a sex difference which has been demonstrated for children in general (Hayden, 1989). Finally, female bullies were perceived by peers to be more attractive than male bullies, whereas male bullies were perceived to be more athletic than female bullies–a finding which is not surprising considering prevailing gender-role stereotypes. The characteristics associated with bullying were also found to differ significantly across the elementary and secondary school contexts. Consistent with research on the development of aggression (see Bjorkqvist, Lagerspetz, & Kaukiainen, 1992), a decrease in the use of physical aggression (for male bullies) with increased age was noted, as was a decrease in the use of relational aggression (for female and male bullies) with increased age.

In the present study, we saw that bullying was associated with both explicit and implicit forms of social power (LaFreniere & Charlesworth, 1983). Bullies were generally perceived to be physically and relationally aggressive, both of which are classic forms of explicit power over others and at least some bullies were also perceived to be leaders and to possess certain non-behavioral competencies and assets that are valued in the peer group, including wealth, attractiveness, and/or athletic competence, which more aptly suggests implicit power. These generally positive correlates of bullying were not enjoyed by all bullies, however. Three subgroups of bullies were distinguished on the basis of their relative power within the group, as perceived by peers. The fact that over half of the students who were identified as bullies were categorized as *powerful* bullies, and only a few (14%) were categorized as relatively powerless is indeed noteworthy. Powerful bullies, in contrast to moderate power bullies and low power bullies, were perceived by peers to possess a mixture of both positive and negative characteristics which, as predicted, reflect both explicit and implicit sources of social power (LaFreniere & Charlesworth, 1983). Powerful bullies were viewed as more popular and more liked as well as more physically and relationally aggressive than less powerful bullies. Additionally, consistent with the notion of implicit power, powerful bullies were perceived to possess more competencies and assets than less powerful bullies, including such things as being physically attractive, wearing stylish clothing, and being better leaders. Although we believe that leadership and peer-valued characteristics are at the core of implicit social power, we also recognize the need for more direct measures of this form of power. For example, future research on implicit power would benefit from asking students questions such as, "Who do you look up to?" or "Who do you want to be like?" that would also reflect a recognition of status and competence.

Contrary to expectations, no statistically significant differences across bully subtypes were found on social self-perceptions or self-reported internalizing difficulties. Why might this be the case? It is possible that, generally speaking, oppressing others feels good and this positive feeling is not dependent upon one's level of peer perceived power. Interestingly, the growing consensus in the self-esteem literature is that individuals with high self-esteem are the ones who aggress when there is a threat to ego as opposed to those with low self-esteem (see Baumeister, Smart, & Boden, 1996 for a review). It is also possible that differences were not found across bully subtypes because bullies (and power) were identified using peer nominations as opposed to self-reports. As such, it could be that bullies are not even aware of their level of power within the peer group, nor may they be aware that they are perceived as bullies by their peers. This lack of awareness of how the peer group views them may be why their social self-perceptions and self-reported internalizing difficulties did not differ across varying levels of perceived power. These points notwithstanding, it is important to consider that the correlation patterns obtained in this study suggest that both powerful students and bullies by and large feel good about themselves and their social interactions.

The present results replicate previous findings that bullies are generally rejected/disliked (e.g., Boulton, 1999; Boulton & Smith, 1994; Pelligrini et al., 1999), but also confirm our expectations that, for a significant number of bullies, bullying behavior is associated with a high degree of social status. As hypothesized, greater power was evident among bullies who utilized both "explicit power" and "implicit power." Perhaps as a result of these characteristics, powerful bullies were more likely to be viewed as popular, despite the fact that they were significantly more physically and relationally aggressive toward peers than their less powerful counterparts. In this regard, this research joins with a growing number of studies suggesting that bullying and other forms of aggressive behavior can be used to enhance and maintain one's status within the peer group (e.g., Espelage & Holt, in press).

Implications for School-Based Intervention Strategies

In considering the implications of these findings for school-based efforts to reduce bullying, it is important to highlight that over half of the students identified by peers as bullies in the present study actually enjoyed a substantial level of status and power within the adolescent peer group, and some were even well liked. The relatively high status enjoyed by most bullies, as well as their recognized positive qualities (e.g., leadership, athletic competence) may in part account for why teachers are able to accurately identify fewer than half of the bullies identified by peers (Leff, Kupersmidt, Patterson, & Power, 1999). Perhaps the fact that many high status bullies display a number of positive characteristics is one reason why teachers, as well as peers, seem to overlook, dismiss, or give them the "benefit of the doubt" with regard to their negative social behavior. Teachers and other adults need to become more aware of the bullying behavior that is perpetrated and possibly legitimized when engaged in by high status students.

A second, but equally important, implication of the present findings concerns the likelihood of changing such behaviors. Indeed, convincing popular students to reduce bullying behavior will be difficult, if not impossible, when such behavior is viewed as a source of privilege, power, and/or status among peers, and when the status afforded them leads them to view their social interactions as effective and successful (see Hughes, Cavell, & Grossman, 1999; regarding aggressive children). This point is particularly true if we consider that being popular and dominant are important pursuits in adolescence (Gavin & Furman, 1989), and that adolescents actually admire aggressive peers (Bukowski, Sippola, & Newcomb, 2000). Zero-tolerance policies and other school-based programs that strive to reduce bullying by establishing negative sanctions against such behavior may be inadequate to counter the status and apparent social "success" associated with such behavior among powerful bullies. High status and powerful bullies may be particularly resistant to change if they perceive their social interactions to be socially accepted, as well as instrumental.

In this regard, it is important to underscore the generally positive self-perceptions expressed by bullies in the present study. Olweus (e.g., 1993) has long argued that bullies do not lack self-esteem. The present results both replicate and extend these findings by demonstrating that positive self-perceptions are evident across several self-report indices and by offering some suggestions regarding *why* this might be the case. Research on the development of children's self-perceptions of competence across domains (Hymel, LeMare, Ditner, & Woody, 1999) indicates that children's *social* self-perceptions are derived largely from their subjective interpretations of how they are treated within the peer group. Relative to other domains in which more objective information regarding performance is available (e.g., academic test scores, grades), the social "feedback" individuals receive is largely ambiguous and difficult to verify (Bohrnstedt & Felson, 1983), but nevertheless constitutes the primary "data base" on which students base their social self-perceptions. Our results suggest that the feedback provided to bullies by the peer group is largely positive, as peers consider these students to be popular and powerful and acknowledge their positive qualities (e.g., appearance, athletic competence), despite their aggressive behavior. As we have argued elsewhere with regard to the social self-perceptions of aggressive-rejected children (e.g., Hymel, Bowker, & Woody, 1993), such positive peer feedback and treatment make it difficult for bullies to recognize the negative aspects of their behavior and instead contributes to positive perceptions of their own social situation, making it difficult to recognize the need for behavior change. In short, it will be difficult to convince powerful bullies that such behavior is without its own rewards. Similarly, for those students who engage in bullying but do *not* enjoy high levels of status and power among their peers, these powerful bullies may serve as models for the potential "success" of such behavior within the school peer group.

Finally, the fact that bullying is common among high status and powerful peers also has implications for efforts to enlist the aid of peer bystanders in reducing bullying behavior. Bullying is increasingly recognized as a group phenomenon that can be fully addressed only when one considers the group processes that operate (e.g., Salmivalli, 1999). Indeed, Hazler (1996) argues that peers are a critical, but largely untapped resource in school-based anti-bullying efforts. Support for such arguments comes from observational studies that indicate that bullying is an underground activity that adults often miss, although peers are present during most bully-victim episodes (e.g., 85-88% of the time), although they seldom intervene on behalf of victims (i.e., 11-19% of the time; e.g., Craig & Pepler, 1995, 1997). In fact, Craig and Pepler (1995) found that peers actually reinforce the bully in about 81% of the episodes and are more respectful and more amiable toward the bully than the victim following such episodes. Although most students reported that they disapproved of bullies' behavior, Salmivalli and Voeten (2002) found that the majority did nothing to help the victim of such attacks, and that 20-30% of children actually encourage the bully, even to the point of joining in (Pepler, 2001). Obviously, such peer responses serve to encourage rather than discourage bullying behavior.

The present results provide some insight into how peer group dynamics can serve to *reduce* the likelihood of peer interventions on behalf of victims. First, confronting a high status and powerful bully may be particularly difficult for more marginal or less powerful members of the peer group. Consistent with these arguments is evidence to suggest that when bystanders *do* intervene on behalf of the victim, such behavior is typically undertaken only by students with high social status (e.g., Salmivalli, Lagerpetz, Bjorkqvist, Osterman, & Kaukiainen, 1996). If only high status peers are likely to be successful in intervening on the part of the victim, perhaps they should be targeted in school-based intervention efforts. Second, supporting a victim carries considerable risk for loss of social status if the bully is both popular and powerful within the group. For most students, it may be more socially advantageous to support the more powerful and high status bully. If so, school-based, anti-bullying programs, especially those that encourage peer bystanders to intervene, will be difficult to implement. Such programs can be effective only if the peer group does not empower the bully by revering and supporting him or her. The fact that over half of the bullies in the present sample were viewed as high status (popular) and powerful makes peer support to such aggressors difficult to eliminate.

The present results underscore the need for a broader and more ecologically valid approach to the problem of bullying in schools, addressing characteristics of the individual, the family, school and community context in which he or she lives (see Swearer & Doll, in press). The present results also support Sutton, Smith, and Swettenham's (1999) arguments for a reconsideration of our deficit-based model of social difficulties, recognizing that many bullies actually demonstrate rather effective and well-developed social skills. By understanding the positive social functions that bullying and other forms of aggressive behavior serve (e.g., Ollendick, 1996; Prinstein, & Cillessen, in press), we may begin to develop more effective and valid approaches to intervention.

NOTE

1. Unlimited nominations have been found to yield sociometric scores with superior distributional properties (i.e., less skewed, wider range of scores) than the more traditional limited (3-5) nomination procedures (see Terry, 2000).

REFERENCES

Adler, P.A. & Adler, P. (1998). *Peer power: Preadolescent culture and identity.* NY: Rutgers University Press.

Asher, S.R., Hymel, S., & Renshaw, P.D. (1984). Loneliness in children. *Child Development, 55,* 1456-1464.

Baumeister, R., Smart, L., & Boden, J. (1996). Relation of threatened egotism to violence and aggression: The dark side of high self-esteem. *Psychological Review, 103,* 5-33.

Besag, V.E. (1989). Bullies and victims in schools. Philadelphia: Open University Press.

Bjorkqvist, K., Lagerspetz, K.M.J., & Kaukiainen, A. (1992). Do girls manipulate and boys fight? Developmental trends in regard to direct and indirect aggression. *Aggressive Behavior, 18,* 117-127.

Bohrnstedt, G.W. & Felson, R.B. (1983). Explaining the relations among children's actual and perceived performances and self-esteem: A comparison of several causal models. *Journal of Personality and Social Psychology, 45,* 43-56.

Boulton, M.J. (1999). Concurrent and longitudinal relations between children's playground behavior and social preference, victimization, and bullying. *Child Development, 70,* 944-954.

Boulton, M.J. & Smith, P.K. (1994). Bully/victim problems in middle-school children: Stability, self-perceived competence, peer perceptions and peer acceptance. *British Journal of Development Psychology, 12,* 315-329.

Bukowski, W.M., Sippola, L.K., & Newcomb, A.F. (2000). Variations in patterns of attraction to same- and other-sex peers during adolescence. *Developmental Psychology, 36,* 147-154.

Coie, J.D. & Dodge, K.A. (1983). Continuities and change in children's social status: A five-year longitudinal study. *Merrill-Palmer Quarterly, 29,* 261-282.

Coie, J.D. & Dodge, K.A. (1998). Aggression and antisocial behavior. In W. Damon (Series Ed.) and N. Eisenberg (Vol. Ed.), *Handbook of child psychology: Vol. 3, Social emotional and personality development* (5th edition, pp. 779-862). NY: Wiley.

Craig, W.M. & Pepler, D.J. (1995). Peer processes in bullying and victimization: An observational study. *Exceptionality Education Canada, 5,* 81-95.

Craig, W.M. & Pepler, D.J. (1997). Observations of bullying and victimization in the schoolyard. *Canadian Journal of School Psychology, 13,* 41-60.

Crick, N.R. & Grotpeter, J.K. (1995). Relational aggression, gender and social-psychological adjustment. *Child Development, 66,* 710-722.

Espelage, D.L. & Holt, M.K. (in press). Bullying and victimization in early adolescence: Peer influences and psychosocial correlates. *Journal of Emotional Abuse.*

Estell, D.B., Cairns, R.B., Farmer, T.W., & Cairns, B.D. (2002). Aggression in inner-city early elementary classrooms: Individual and peer-group configurations. *Merrill-Palmer Quarterly, 48,* 52-76.

Farmer, T.W. & Rodkin, P.C. (1996). Antisocial and prosocial correlates of social positions: The social network centrality perspective. *Social Development, 5,* 174-188.

Forero, R. & McLellan, L. (1999). Bullying behaviour and psychosocial health among school students in New South Wales, Australia. *British Medical Journal, 319,* 344-348.

Galen, B.R. & Underwood, M.K. (1997). A developmental investigation of social aggression among children. *Developmental Psychology, 33,* 589-600.

Gavin, L.A. & Furman, W. (1989). Age differences in adolescents' perceptions of their peer groups. *Developmental Psychology, 25,* 1-8.

Hayden, L.K. (1989). *Children's loneliness.* Unpublished doctoral dissertation, University of Waterloo, Waterloo, Ontario, Canada.

Hazler, R.J. (1996). Bystanders: An overlooked factor in peer on peer abuse. *Journal for the Professional Counselor, 11,* 11-21.

Hess, L.E. & Atkins, M.S. (1998). Victims and aggressors at school: Teachers, self, and peer perceptions of psychosocial functioning. *Applied Developmental Science, 2,* 75-89.

Hughes, J.H., Cavell, T.A., & Grossman, P.B. (1997). A positive view of self: Risk or protection for aggressive children? *Development and Psychopathology, 9,* 75-94.

Hymel, S., Bowker, A., & Woody, E. (1993). Aggressive versus withdrawn unpopular children: Variations in peer and self-perceptions in multiple domains. *Child Development, 64,* 879-896.

Hymel, S., LeMare, L., Ditner, E., & Woody, E.Z. (1999). Assessing self-concept in children: Variations across self-concept domains. *Merrill Palmer Quarterly, 45,* 602-623.

Kaltiala-Heino, R., Rimpela, M., Marttunen, M., Rimpela, A., & Rantanen, P. (1999). Bullying, depression and suicidal ideation in Finnish adolescents: School survey. *British Medical Journal, 319,* 348-351.

Kovacs, M. (1991/1992). *Children's Depression Inventory Manual.* Multi Health Systems, Inc.: Toronto.

Kumpulainen, K., Rasanen, E., Henttonen, I., Almqvist, F., Kresanov, K., Linna, S., Moilanen, I., Piha, J., Purra, K., & Tamminen, T. (1998). Bullying and psychiatric symptoms among elementary school-age children. *Child Abuse and Neglect, 22,* 705-717.

LaFreniere, P. & Charlesworth, W.R. (1983). Dominance, attention, and affiliation in a preschool group: A nine-month longitudinal study. *Ethology and Sociobiology, 4,* 55-67.

Leff, S.S., Kupersmidt, J.B., Patterson, C.J., & Power, T.J. (1999). Factors influencing teacher identification of peer bullies and victims. *School Psychology Review, 28,* 505-517.

Marsh, H. (1988). *Self-Description Questionnaire I Manual.* Harcourt Brace Jovanovich, Inc.: Toronto.

Merten, D.E. (1997). The meaning of meanness: Popularity, competition, and conflict among junior high school girls. *Sociology of Education, 70,* 175-191.

Nansel, T.R., Overpeck, M., Pilla, R.S., Ruan, W. J., Simons-Morton, B., & Scheidt, P. (2001). Bullying behaviors among US youth: Prevalence and association with psychosocial adjustment. *Journal of the American Medical Association (JAMA), 285,* 2094-2100.

Ollendick, T.H. (1996). Violence in youth: Where do we go from here? Behavior Therapy's response. *Behavior Therapy, 27,* 485-514.

Olweus, D. (1973). *Hackkycklingar och oversittare. Forskning om skolmobbning.* Stockholm: Almqvist & Wicksell.

Olweus, D. (1978). *Aggression in schools: Bullies and whipping boys.* Washington, DC: Hemisphere.

Olweus, D. (1993). *Bullying in school: What we know and what we can do.* Oxford: Blackwell.

Olweus, D. (1994). Annotation: Bullying at school: Basic facts and effects of a school based intervention program. *Journal of Child Psychology & Psychiatry & Allied Disciplines, 35,* 1171-1190.

Olweus, D. (1996). Bullying at school: Knowledge base and an effective intervention program. In C.F. Ferris & T. Grisso (Eds.), *Understanding aggressive behavior in children. Annals of the New York Academy of Sciences, Vol. 794* (pp. 265-276). NY: New York Academy of Sciences.

Parkhurst, J.T. & Hopmeyer, A. (1998). Sociometric popularity and peer-perceived popularity: Two distinct dimensions of peer status. *Journal of Early Adolescence, 18,* 125-144.

Pellegrini, A.D., Bartini, M., & Brooks, F. (1999). School bullies, victims, and aggressive victims: Factors relating to group affiliation and victimization in early adolescence. *Journal of Educational Psychology, 91,* 216-224.

Pepler, D. (2001, May). Peer group dynamics and the culture of violence. In S. Hymel (Chair), Culture of violence. Paper symposium for the annual meeting of the Royal Society of Canada (Academy II) and the Canadian Society for Studies in Education, Quebec.

Perry, D.G., Kusel, S.J., & Perry, L.C. (1988). Victims of peer aggression. *Developmental Psychology, 24,* 807-814.

Prinstein, M.J. & Cillessen, A.H.N. (2003). Forms and functions of adolescent peer aggression associated with high levels of peer status. *Merrill-Palmer Quarterly, 49,* 30-342.

Rigby, K. (1999). Peer victimization at school and the health of secondary school students. *British Journal of Educational Psychology, 69,* 95-104.

Rolan, E. (2002). Aggression, depression and bullying others. *Aggressive Behavior, 28,* 198-2002.

Rubin, K.H., Bukowski, W. & Parker, J.G. (1998). Peer interactions, relationships and groups. In W. Damon (Series Ed.) and N. Eisenberg (Vol. Ed.), *Handbook of child psychology: Vol. 3, Social emotional and personality development* (5th edition, pp. 619-700). NY: Wiley.

Salmivalli, C. (1999). Participant role approach to school bullying: Implications for interventions. *Journal of Adolescence, 22,* 453-459.

Salmivalli, C., Lagerspetz, K., Bjorkqvist, K., Osterman, K., & Kaukiainen, A. (1996). Bullying as a group process: Participant roles and their relations to social status within the group. *Aggressive Behavior, 22,* 1-15.

Salmivalli, C. & Voeten, M. (2002). Connections between attitudes, group norms, and behavior in bullying situations. Manuscript submitted for publication.

Schwartz, D. (2000). Subtypes of victims and aggressors in children's peer groups. *Journal of Abnormal Child Psychology, 28,* 181-192.

Sletta, O. (1998). *Social Self-Efficacy Scale for Adolescents.* Unpublished scale.

Sutton, J. & Smith, P.K. (1999). Bullying as a group process: An adaptation of the participant role approach. *Aggressive Behavior, 25,* 97-111.

Swearer, S.M. & Doll, B. (in press). Bullying in schools: An ecological framework. *Journal of Emotional Abuse.*

Terrell-Deutsch, B. (1999). The conceptualization and measurement of childhood loneliness. In K.J. Rotenberg and S. Hymel (Eds.), *Loneliness in childhood and adolescence* (pp. 11-33). New York: Cambridge University Press.

Terry, R. (2000). Recent advances in measurement theory and the use of sociometric techniques. In A.H.N. Cillessen & W.M. Bukowski (Eds.), *Recent advances in the study and measurement of acceptance and rejection in the peer system. New Directions for Child Development* (No. 88). CA: Jossey-Bass.

Vaillancourt, T. & Hymel, S. (2002). Understanding sociometric status: What does it mean to be popular? Manuscript submitted for publication.

Wheeler, V.A. & Ladd, G.W. (1982). Assessment of children's self-efficacy for social interactions with peers. *Developmental Psychology, 18,* 795-805.

Sexual Harassment
and the Cultures of Childhood:
Developmental, Domestic Violence,
and Legal Perspectives

Philip C. Rodkin
Karla Fischer
University of Illinois at Urbana-Champaign

SUMMARY. Sexual harassment is increasingly recognized as a common problem for schoolchildren. Four out of five 8th through 11th graders have experienced some form of sexual harassment in their school lives. Of the girls who experience harassment, 38% report that they were first harassed in 6th grade or before (AAUW, 2001). We propose that children construct a peer-based "school society" where attitudes and behaviors are strongly connected to peer group influence and concerns

Address correspondence to either: Philip C. Rodkin, 220B Education Building, Mail Code 708, Department of Educational Psychology, University of Illinois at Urbana-Champaign, 1310 S. 6th Street, Champaign, IL 61820. Karla Fischer, College of Law, Mail Code 594, University of Illinois at Urbana-Champaign, 504 E. Pennsylvania Avenue, Champaign, IL 61820 (E-mail: kfischer@aw.uiuc.edu) or (E-mail: kfischer@law.uiuc.edu) or (E-mail: rodkin@uiuc.edu).

This work was supported by a Faculty Fellows grant from the Bureau of Educational Research, College of Education, University of Illinois at Urbana-Champaign to Philip C. Rodkin.

[Haworth co-indexing entry note]: "Sexual Harassment and the Cultures of Childhood: Developmental, Domestic Violence, and Legal Perspectives." Rodkin, Philip C., and Karla Fischer. Co-published simultaneously in *Journal of Applied School Psychology* (The Haworth Press, Inc.) Vol. 19, No. 2, 2003, pp. 177-196; and: *Bullying, Peer Harassment, and Victimization in the Schools: The Next Generation of Prevention* (ed: Maurice J. Elias, and Joseph E. Zins) The Haworth Press, Inc., 2003, pp. 177-196. Single or multiple copies of this article are available for a fee from The Haworth Document Delivery Service [1-800-HAWORTH, 9:00 a.m. - 5:00 p.m. (EST). E-mail address: docdelivery@haworthpress.com].

10.1300/J008v19n02_11

about social status. School-based peer sexual harassment emerges from a climate of tense, unequal social relations between boys and girls during middle childhood, accelerating into adolescence. One unexplored possibility is that some boys with high social status among their peers may engage in or encourage harassment of girls. Next, we turn to a distinct social context embedded within the school society: relationships of abuse between boy and girl peers. We explore how the dynamics of domestic violence apply to sexual harassment between peers, illustrating themes from narratives of child sexual harassment victims derived from interviews and legal cases. We also use these narratives to examine the institutional responses to sexual harassment by school authorities, identifying the parallels to domestic violence legal solutions. Our discussion emphasizes how school service providers can better appreciate and react to the social and relational context of boys' harassment of girls. *[Article copies available for a fee from the Haworth Document Delivery Service: 1-800-HAWORTH. E-mail address: <docdelivery@haworthpress.com> Website: <http://www.HaworthPress.com> © 2003 by The Haworth Press, Inc. All rights reserved.]*

KEYWORDS. Sexual harassment, domestic violence, peer relations, middle childhood, social status

Communities of children both reflect and transform into communities of adults, so it should come as little surprise when the pathologies of one generation are also manifested in the other. Sexual harassment, once thought to be a social problem exclusive to women in the workplace, is now recognized as a common experience for both girls and boys in school. As revealed by the AAUW's well-known *Hostile Hallways* surveys, four out of five 8th through 11th graders have experienced some form of sexual harassment in their school lives (AAUW, 1993, 2001). Sexual harassment is an intimidating challenge for school service providers, who have just begun to scratch the surface of the too-often aggressive, coercive, destructive behavior patterns between boys and girls in the early adolescent years. The repercussions of school-based harassment are severe: harassment leads to children staying home from school, not talking as much in class, and decreasing their attention to their classwork (AAUW, 1993). For girls, harassment has additional detriments, most prominently to their self-esteem (Murnen & Smolak, 2001). Despite the serious effects of sexual harassment, teachers and school officials often downplay its significance: sometimes by looking the other way, other times by standing by as girls are harassed in front of them in the school corridors and even the classrooms (Phillips, 1998). This "head in the sand" approach has earned school districts wide condemnation in the courts as well as legal liability (Romano, 2001). Threatened with large, punitive consequences, school service providers have promoted quick, sometimes drastic, and not necessarily optimal educational responses to the larger issue of how boys and girls relate to one another.

According to the AAUW report (2001, p. 2), sexual harassment is: "unwanted and unwelcome sexual behavior that interferes with your life. Sexual harassment is not behaviors that you like or want (for example, wanted kissing, touching, or flirting)." At its core, peer sexual harassment is about aggressive and power-based social interactions between boys and girls. Because aggression and power are conjoined in many situations, we look to two arenas closely related to peer sexual harassment that help illuminate common issues and their solutions. First, we describe how aggression can sometimes fit naturally into elementary and middle school societies, an ecology where interactions between boys and girls are typically negative. Second, we examine the psychological reactions of adult victims to domestic violence and track the institutional responses to reporting. In each case, we attend to the implications of the research for peer sexual harassment. Our larger aim is to objectify social forces that, because they fade invisibly into the normal workings of social ecologies, are easy to overlook (Milgram, 1977; Ross & Nisbett, 1991). Indeed, we feel that adults who deal with peer sexual harassment issues may sometimes fail to recognize critical relational and cultural dynamics that enable harassment to flourish. We attempt to help foster appropriate responses to peer-based sexual harassment that are legally sensitive, responsive to the reality of children's gendered social development, and cognizant of the social supports that promote a culture of negativity between boys and girls in childhood and early adolescence. Our primary concern here is with the phenomenon of boys harassing girls, as this is not only the most common form of harassment, but also the most severe in terms of psychological consequences (Romano, 2001).

DEVELOPMENTAL PERSPECTIVES: GENDER, AGGRESSION, AND STATUS IN CHILDREN'S SCHOOL SOCIETIES

Our interpretation of research on children's social development is that peer-based sexual harassment: (a) has its origins in the gendered peer cultures of early and middle childhood, and (b) is propelled forward by peer culture norms, to which both boys and girls may contribute, that legitimizes at least some kinds of aggression for some boys. Could boys' harassment of girls be a peer-sanctioned form of aggression? The question is unanswered in current research, but the hypothesis needs to be explored. We hope that our review can give some guidance to those interested in how the interpersonal dynamic of peer sexual harassment might be conceptualized, and in how to focus prevention and intervention attempts.

Developmental origins: The school societies of middle childhood. We begin with a conceptual heuristic called the *school society*. The school society framework is a structuralist-agentic form of a more general class of contextual-holistic theories (e.g., Cairns, Elder, & Costello, 1996; Farmer, 2000) that view social behavior as a joint product of a person acting within his or her subjective social environment (Coleman, 1961; Lewin, 1943). A social environment is not a unitary place, nor can it be assessed with a single measure. Rather, social environments are multileveled and characterized by hierarchical micro- to macrosocial structures (e.g., peer social network, classroom, school, community, national culture) that Bronfenbrenner (1979, p. 3) "conceived as a set of nested structures, each inside the next, like a set of Russian dolls." The strongest contextual elicitors of behavior are the proximal, microsocial situations in which behavior unfolds. The right proximal contexts to examine depend upon the kind of behavior under study and the setting (e.g., school, home) in which it occurs. For example, as children make the transition from elementary to middle or junior high school the classroom (but not the peer group or school) often (but not always) loses its coherence as a meaningful social unit.

The school society heuristic focuses specifically on peer interaction in school-based settings. Other, larger social contexts, such as media influences on society or national policy, can frame the culture of the school society from a top-down perspective but are often removed from children's day-to-day interactions with one another. The most prominent social structures in the school society organize children's behavior–and here we focus on children's gendered and/or aggressive behavior–horizontally and vertically. By *horizontally*, we mean that even simple grade school classrooms are contoured social environments featuring multiple *peer groups* (i.e., cliques) and hence multiple avenues for children to find a niche and mobilize social support. Peer groups are microsocial structures. They include a small number of children (e.g., two or three to seven or eight) and are often the most immediate context of children's perceptions and behaviors (Allen, 1981; Cairns, Xie, & Leung, 1998). Children inevitably construct distinct (but also dynamic and overlapping) peer groups that are segregated by gender, race and ethnicity (see Graham & Juvonen, 2002), and other demographic and behavioral attributes. Our emphasis on the group as the seminal unit of the school society falls closely in line with Kurt Lewin (1943, p. 115), who wrote that "all education is group work."

By *vertical structure*, we mean that children and their peer groups vary in *social status and influence*. The vertical structure of the school society corresponds to a dimension of social power (cf., Lippitt, Polansky, Redl, & Rosen, 1952) and is usually accepted by children as a source of legitimate peer authority even when it is personally disliked. One important consequence of social status differences is that some children have more of a say than others in determining what their peers value and devalue, support and stigmatize. When considering aggressive behavior, particularly boys' aggression toward girls, this perspective broadens the focus from the well-established connection between aggression and low social status (e.g., peer rejection) to include recent findings showing that aggression and social status can be positively related (e.g., Rodkin, Farmer, Pearl, & van Acker, 2000). For the school psychologist, this boils down to a question of whether the underlying dynamics of a harassment episode(s) lies in the margins or nearer to the heart of the dominant peer cultures.

Structuralist accounts of social environments like the school society can often seem static, but descriptions and explanations of peer sexual harassment need to be developmentally oriented. Developmental trajectories are important to examine over both the short term and the long term. By *short-term trajectories*, we focus on events that occur over the course of a school year or two that can yield insight into the formation, stabilization—and sometimes alteration—of a school society. The most elegant analyses of short-term developmental changes have involved studies of children's social interaction at summer camp (Lippitt et al., 1952; Parker & Seal, 1996; Sherif, 1956). For example, in the Robbers Cave experiments with white, 11- and 12-year-olds, Sherif (1956) tracked in fascinating detail the natural formation of peer groups and social hierarchies, their later consolidation into deeply entrenched, intensely negative intergroup dynamics, and finally their radical alteration from aggression to collaboration by outside intervention. Developments over the short term are essential for explaining the norms and interpersonal dynamics that arise within a school society, but they have been largely overlooked in recent literature. Instead, researchers have focused on *long-term trajectories* where focus is on how behavior patterns that are established during one stage of the life course (e.g., middle childhood) set children on paths towards adjustment or maladjustment in adolescence and beyond. For example, researchers whose interest lies primarily in predicting which boys will go on to become serious abusers as men would concentrate on long-term developmental trajectories.

What are the implications of a school society framework for sexual harassment? Peer groups and social status are critical elements of the interpersonal context between harassers and victims. AAUW (2001, p. 41) reports that four in ten self-reported harassers defend their actions by saying that "a lot of people do it" and one-quarter "say their friends encouraged or pushed them to do it" (multiple responses were possible so percentages are not exclusive). These answers implicate others in the harasser's environment and call for a framework where we know how harassers are socially connected to their peers. Harassment is often a group activity (AAUW, 2001, p. 26) and as the literature on children's bullying suggests (reviewed below), it often occurs under group influence. Thanks to the presence of multiple social groups (i.e., centers of influence), school societies like most societies tolerate multiple, dissonant messages. Many children may be in prominent peer groups that promote and accept dominant societal values. But other children may be in equally prominent peer groups (prominent, at least, to other children) that promote subversive messages of aggression and harassment. As we describe later in our paper, in many sexual harassment cases school officials seemed to fail to recognize these subversive groups, with adults intentionally or unintentionally supporting negative peer group attitudes about gender. Childhood social status is closely aligned with the values of peer culture, where those with more status have a greater say in generating the values of the group. Neither childhood nor adult sexual harassment could ever be understood without a concept of power in the equation. The dominant framework for childhood social status in the developmental literature focuses on likeability, not power or prominence, and so the possibility that popular leaders in peer cultures could engage in sexual harassment has not been a focus.

Gender boundaries and borderwork in school societies. Even though peer sexual harassment may take on more recognizable (i.e., adult) forms during the dramatic transition to adolescence (e.g., AAUW, 1993, 2001; Craig, Pepler, Connolly, & Henderson, 2001), dysfunctional interaction patterns between boys and girls take root in middle childhood. The 2001 AAUW survey (p. 25) reports that 38% of girls who experience sexual harassment "say they first experienced it in elementary school: sixth grade or before." Eleanor Maccoby's (1998) book *The Two Sexes* makes three critical points on the origins of negative boy-girl interactions. First, children's preference for same-sex peers emerges between two to three years of age (with girls exhibiting same-sex preferences somewhat before boys) and consolidates during the grade school years. Second, gender differentiation requires the continued presence of children's peer groups, the horizontal structure of school societies. Third, Maccoby points out that the active ingredient in children's gendered social development is the children themselves. Children actively construct separate cultures of male and female peer groups in which interaction with opposite-sex peers (henceforth *opposite-sex interaction*) becomes uneasy and tense. Parents and educators may validate negative opposite-sex interactions, going along with children's constructions of gender rather than resisting its negative excesses, or trying to alter (as difficult as it may be) normative developmental trajectories of behavior towards opposite-sex peers.

Recent research supports the Maccoby thesis. Gender segregation is quite possibly the signature phenomenon of middle childhood social development. A number of studies have found that the internal structure of boys' and girls' groups differ from one another, with boys' groups being larger, more cohesive, and more stratified on the basis of power and status (Benenson, Apostoleris, & Parnass, 1998). Boy and girl peer groups can also diverge on the behavioral and social characteristics that children support and emulate. Groups of boys tend to value toughness and competition, while for girls material possessions, cooperation and intimacy, and physical appearance may have the strongest links to social status (Adler & Adler, 1998; Maccoby, 1998).

The portrait drawn so far suggests that boys and girls choose to affiliate in starkly gender segregated peer groups. Boys and girls in middle childhood, despite being in the same classroom, live in psychologically "separate" (Thorne, 1993) or "special" (Bernard, 1979) worlds with few opportunities for voluntary interaction. But even strong boundaries are permeable. As two cultures living in close proximity within the confines of a larger social unit (i.e., the classroom or school), intergroup dynamics inevitably develop. Maccoby (1998) suggests that groups of boys and girls do not merely differ in a separate-but-equal fashion, but that there also exists an entrenched power asymmetry in favor of boys. Social development research increasingly indicates that opposite-sex interaction, called "borderwork" by Thorne (1993), too often constitutes a zone of danger for female students–a highly charged, uncomfortable, unbalanced, ill-defined affiliative zone (Adler & Adler, 1998; Eder, Evans, & Parker, 1995; Maccoby, 1998).

The study of children's enemies is a newly emerging body of work that has potential to shed significant light on social relationships between boys and girls (Hodges & Card, in press). Enemy relationships have typically been measured by asking children to nominate peers whom they "like least" or "would least like as a play or work partner" and identifying reciprocated, mutual nominations of dislike (i.e., A nominates B as "liked least" and B returns the favor). Rodkin, Pearl, Farmer, and van Acker (in press) examined the nature of children's enemy relationships in a mostly suburban sample of approximately 500 children followed from the spring of 3rd grade to the spring of 4th grade. They examined the proportion of enemy dyads that were composed of a boy and a girl, two boys, and two girls. One possibility, following from a strong form of the "separate worlds" hypothesis was that boys and girls would rarely name one another as enemies for the same reason that they rarely nominate one another as friends–that a buffer zone of neutrality, ignorance, and lack of awareness exists between the sexes. Instead, 52% of enemy dyads in the spring of 3rd grade were between boys and girls, with only a slightly smaller rate of opposite-sex enemies (41-42%) during the two 4th grade assessments.

Other studies also show that opposite-sex enmities are common in middle childhood and early adolescence (Abecassis, Hartup, Haselager, Scholte, & van Lieshout, 2002; Hodges & Card, in press). Sometimes, enmity between a boy and a girl may be the only legitimate way to express any feelings towards a member of the opposite sex, including feelings of sexual tension or interest (Adler & Adler, 1998, p. 166; Maccoby, 1998, p. 69). Other times, opposite-sex enmities may reflect a polluted social dynamic between the sexes. For example, Underwood, Schockner, and Hurley (2001) placed 8-, 10-, and 12-year-olds from urban areas of the Pacific Northwest in an experimental scenario where they were teased by either a same- or opposite-sex confederate while losing at a computer game. Observational data indicated that children who were teased by an opposite- as compared to same-sex peer showed more negative facial expressions, made more negative remarks, and displayed more negative gestures. Post-experimental interviews revealed that children liked and wanted to be friends with the provocateur less when they were of the opposite sex.

In sum, we propose that boys' harassment of girls emerges from and can be elicited by a climate of tense, unequal social relations between groups of boys and groups of girls beginning in middle childhood. Indeed, mutual antipathy may be one of the only kinds of relationships that indexes borderwork between boys and girls at school. Of course, social environments do not, in and of themselves, cause any one boy to sexually harass any one girl. We turn now to the vertical structure of school societies, focusing on prevailing social norms toward at least some forms of male aggression (e.g., proactive, instrumental) and the characteristics of boys held in high status among their peers. Our review will speculate that at least some high status boys and/or their affiliates may be particularly effective at sexually harassing opposite-sex peers. More generally, norms that support aggressive behavior can be pervasive and need to be an important area in future peer relations and peer sexual harassment research.

Relations between social status and aggression among boys. More than one school psychologist has told us that their professional training led them to expect that popular children would be prosocial and aggressive children would be rejected, until their professional experiences proved otherwise. Ethnographers of children's peer culture were among the first to conclude that popular elementary (Adler & Adler, 1998) and middle school (Eder et al., 1995; Merten, 1997) children, whether male or female, could be rebellious, ruthless, and Machiavellian in establishing and maintaining their high social positions (see Rodkin et al. (2000) for a more extensive review). Rodkin et al. (2000) examined subtypes of popular 4th to 6th grade boys in a diverse sample of urban and rural children. Popular-prosocial ("model") boys were perceived as cool, athletic, leaders, cooperative, studious, not shy, and nonaggressive, while popular-antisocial ("tough") boys were perceived as cool, athletic, and anti-social. Rodkin et al.'s (2000) findings suggested that highly aggressive boys (if they are also attractive and/or athletic) can be among the most popular and socially connected children in elementary classrooms. In fact, educators should know that aggressive children vary widely in social status (see Farmer, 2000). Rodkin et al.'s (2000) basic finding has been replicated in a variety of samples. There is evidence for tough, popular-aggressive boys in 3rd grade, suburban communities (Estell, Farmer, van Acker, Pearl, & Rodkin, in press) and for older adolescent children the connection between popularity and aggression seems to become even stronger (e.g., LaFontana & Cillessen, 2002; Gorman, Kim, & Schimmelbusch, 2002; Prinstein & Cillessen, 2003).

Tough children rely on a network of supporters, subordinates, and scape-goats to establish and exercise influence (Salmivalli, Huttunen, & Lagerspetz, 1997). Recent work suggests that aggressive boys, but less so aggressive girls, are well-established in school societies. Far from being relegated to a low sta-tus, deviant group, 4th to 6th grade aggressive boys affiliate with a wide range of aggressive and nonaggressive peers (Farmer, Leung, Pearl, Rodkin, Cadwallader, & van Acker, 2002). Rodkin (2002) examined whether popu-lar-aggressive boys tended to be nominated as "cool" by a broad or narrow cross-section of their classmates. Results indicated that popular-aggressive boys were peer group leaders, perceived as cool by their fellow group mem-bers, by groups of unpopular boys–and also by girls (see also Bukowski, Sippola, & Newcomb, 2000). The only children not likely to name popular-ag-gressive boys as cool were boys in groups with mostly nonaggressive children. This suggests that popular-aggressive boys have a broad (though not univer-sal) base of support in the elementary classroom to which girls, regardless of their liking for popular-aggressive boys, may contribute.

An emerging literature on bullying and victimization converges closely with research on the popularity of aggression and a school society framework stressing the importance of peer groups and social status. Current research in-dicates that the relationship between bullies and victims involves much of the elementary classroom (O'Connell, Peplar, & Craig, 1999). In a rural sample of 5th graders, bullies tended to be friends with other bullies (Pellegrini, Bartini, & Brooks, 1999). Many children who are not themselves aggressive validate bul-lies with applause, or play supporting roles in bully-led peer groups (O'Connor et al., 1999; Salmivalli et al., 1997). Bullies are often popular within their groups (Pellegrini et al., 1999). Boulton (1999) reported that bullies' cliques tended to be larger than those of non-bullies in an English urban middle school sample of 8- to 12-year-olds. In a 3rd-7th grade mostly white university school sample, Hodges, Malone, and Perry (1997) found that potential victims also rely on a network of supporters that can thwart bullies, but support is only effective if friends are not themselves unpopular or physically weak. These findings have led some to question the traditional view that bullies, as aggressive children, lack social skills and sophistication (Sutton, Smith, & Swettenham, 1999). Indeed, bullies may successfully form a number of distinct relationships with their peers (including the victim him or herself) in order to attain their social goals.

Summary. Children's school societies provide fertile soil for peer sexual harassment. Boys and girls occupy segregated peer groups that promote negative gender stereotypes and relationships of dislike. The leading edge of peer sexual harassment may reside with popular, high status boys, although such a linkage has not been established empirically. One possibility is that popular boys are themselves most likely to, or are at least most effective in, sexually harassing girls. Another possibility is that less popular and/or nonaggressive children in groups dominated by aggressive boys come to believe that harassment is acceptable and status-enhancing. Although our discussion has emphasized conflict between the sexes, middle childhood gender relations can be characterized on multiple dimensions. the agreement between boys and girls on sex-specific aspects of coolness suggests that both boy and girl peer cultures, and the borderwork between them, can work together to contribute to gender socialization. For example, Rodkin's (2002) findings are consistent with Bukowski et al.'s (2000) conclusion that early adolescent girls can become attracted to aggressive boys. Indeed, girls' nominations of tough boys as cool may be the early origins of later attraction to aggressive boys. As Nisbett and Cohen (1996) found in adult, white southern culture, women validate men who aggress over issues of honor to the same extent that men do. Cultural values about aggression may be transmitted to girls even before issues of sexual attraction surface. Any intervention strategy would be wise to attend to these cross-currents of collaboration and competition, enmity and admiration, that flow between boys and girls during childhood and early adolescence.

GENDER AND AGGRESSION IN DOMESTIC VIOLENCE: APPLICATIONS TO PEER SEXUAL HARASSMENT

From our perspective, the most important similarity between peer sexual harassment and domestic violence is that each occurs in complex interpersonal environments marked by the construction of social norms and influence pro-

cesses that can be difficult for outsiders to appreciate. The school society research
sketched out here is a framework for understanding the peer environments within
which relationships of abuse can emerge. Youth culture, increasingly from
middle childhood to adolescence, houses small ecologies that can too easily
engender relationships of abuse. We now turn to an examination of the psycho-
lugical reality of dyadic relationships of abuse, using research on the dynamics
of adult domestic violence as a guide. Once formed, the relationship of abuse
becomes yet another, distinct social context embedded within the school society, even harder for an outsider to penetrate but critical for understanding the
phenomenology of peer sexual harassment and its anchors. As in the social development literature, the literature in domestic violence underscores the importance of power in gendered social interactions. By attending to issues of
power, the domestic violence paradigm offers a relational social context that
complements the school society.

We focus on three ways that domestic violence research may help inform
the problem of sexual harassment between children. First, like adults who are
dating or married to each other, children in classrooms share physical space, a
social environment, and have ongoing relationships. Second, similar to adults
in abusive relationships, sexual harassment between children entails exercises
of control implicating the vertical, power-based structure of classroom societies. Consequently, we might expect to see the same kinds of dynamics between
child sexual harassers and their victims as we do between adult batterers and
their victims. Third, legal responses to domestic violence increasingly build on
the psychological reality of abusive relationships, providing a useful guide for
remedies to childhood sexual harassment. We will identify the sexual harassment dynamics that seem applicable from the domestic violence literature and
illustrate these themes from narratives from child sexual harassment victims
derived from interviews and legal cases. We will suggest that identifying these
dynamics may assist educators in understanding the nature and seriousness of
sexual harassment and, ultimately, in the resolution of disputes in the school
system. Finally, we will examine institutional (legal) responses to domestic violence and their parallels in the response to sexual harassment by school authorities. We close by offering solutions to peer sexual harassment that school
officials can utilize to avoid the problems identified in the domestic violence
literature.

The research on domestic violence that analyzes the dyadic interactions between abuser and abused implicates several common contextual themes that
may apply to sexual harassment between school children in early and mid-ado-
lescence. First, domestic violence abuse is nested within a broader relationship
context of rules and rulemaking, where batterers enforce explicit as well as implicit rules about what victims are and are not allowed to do (Fischer, Vidmar, &

Ellis, 1993). As described in the first part of our paper, a comparable norm-governed context can sometimes be constructed by children in school concerning how girls should and should not be.

Examining the narratives of girls who have been sexually harassed appears to amply support an ongoing rule based culture in schools, with a power asymmetry in favor of boys. This culture sets up a hierarchy of boys controlling girls, and also reinforces a structure in which girls are punished for responding to sexual harassment in active (rather than passive) ways. Similar to domestic violence victims who can explain their relationship rules, girls seem able to articulate the unwritten yet enforced rules in their school. One common rule may be some variation of "the guys would want you to let them touch you all over" (Stein, 1999, p. 15). Girls who refuse to accept this may be threatened or physically assaulted, which serves only to reinforce the rule:

> I could never stand up to him because if I told him to stop he'd threaten me . . . he'd hit me (hard enough to bruise me twice) and then pin my arms behind my back till it hurt and push against a wall and tell me all the awful things he would do to me if I ever hit him again, so I quit standing up to him again.

Some boys who sexually harass girls openly acknowledge power-based reasons for engaging in sexually harassing behavior: because they want dates or something else from their victims (43%) or because they are encouraged or pushed by their friends (20%) (AAUW, 1993). A small percentage of boys (5%) admit that they explicitly wanted their victim to feel less powerful. As with the case of domestic violence, part of the power dynamics between boys and girls in schools may be based on physical size differentials: one of the effects of "anti-bullying" programs may be that boys treat girls differently in terms of global teasing, chasing, and insulting, while girls stop teasing and bullying "shrimpy or short boys" (Stein, 1999, p. 63).

A rule-based school culture, therefore, is more than just the content of the rules (that boys control girls). It is a culture in which sexual harassment is an accepted tool for achieving that control. As Nan Stein (1999) has observed, sexual harassment in schools is public in nature: many incidents of sexual harassment, like the more general instances of bullying described earlier, are not simply between harasser(s) and victim(s), but consist of bystanders and observers–including adult employees of the school. The physical locations of sexual harassment are contained overwhelmingly in the public spaces of schools, the spaces that victims cannot avoid: 65% of sexual harassment takes place in the hallways of the school, while 55% occurs in the classrooms (AAUW,

1993). More than half of all girls who have been harassed report being harassed by a group of boys (AAUW, 1993). The fact that more sexual harassment happens in the public rather than private spaces of schools and in groups rather than in dyads suggests that sexual harassment can become integral to the culture of schools.

Other factors suggest that sexual harassment is well integrated into school culture. Almost half of boys who admit sexually harassing someone (41%) say that they did it because "it's just part of school life" and/or "lots of people do it" (AAUW, 1993); and victims report that experiencing sexual harassment is "normal" and "just one of those things that I have to put up with" (Stein, 1999, p. 146). Many legal cases involving peer harassment, even before *Davis v. Monroe* (giving rise to a cause of action for peer harassment, if school officials know of the conduct but fail to act to stop it) suggest that teachers and principals tend to normalize sexual harassment. For example, in *Bruneau v. South Kortright Central School District* (1996), several girls were verbally harassed in demeaning ways, including being called "lesbian," "whore," and "ugly dog faced bitch." These girls were also physically harassed by these same boys, who snapped their bras, stuffed paper down their blouses, cut their hair, grabbed their breasts, and spit, shoved, hit, and kicked them. When they told one of their teachers about the harassment, he responded that the boys were engaging in "normal flirting and teasing" and that one of the girls "was so beautiful that the boys would be all over her in a couple of years."

If sexual harassment arises from the rule-based cultures of schools, then it is also likely that other domestic violence dynamics are operating in this context. Victims of domestic violence seem to internalize their relationship rules over time by self-censoring their own behavior—altering what they say and what they do. The fact that victims of sexual harassment in schools speak less in class (AAUW, 1993) suggests that self-censoring may be a part of the ongoing power dynamic of the harassment. As the girl in the narrative quoted above expressed, she began to react passively rather than "tell him to stop" to avoid being further harassed. Last, domestic violence victims react in predictable ways to the abuse: because of the shame and embarrassment abuse generates, they hide from others, deny that it is occurring, and minimize its effect. Given that few students tell their teachers (7%) or families (23%) (AAUW, 1993) about the harassment that they have experienced, victims of school-based harassment appear to share the psychological reactions of adult women who have been abused. An important direction for research is to examine these possibilities empirically, elaborating how the domestic violence paradigm aligns with girls' reaction to sexual harassment at school.

Institutional (Legal) Responses to Domestic Violence:
Avoiding Their Pitfalls in Sexual Harassment School Policy

Perhaps it is not surprising that the parallels in the dynamics between peer sexual harassment and domestic violence are similar. A review of the case law in peer sexual harassment suggests striking parallels between institutional responses to domestic violence by legal authorities and institutional responses to sexual harassment by school authorities. Both kinds of authorities have made similar mistakes and fallen into similar pitfalls. In both cases, one avenue for progress is to devise institutional/legal responses that recognize the operating social contexts that support abusive relationships.

As noted earlier, school officials typically respond to victims' complaints of sexual harassment by dismissing it as "normal teasing and flirting" or by failing to react altogether. Now that the Monroe case has opened up the potential for liability by engaging in "head in the sand" approaches to peer harassment, we would expect to see fewer cases of inaction in the future. When school officials do act, however, they often do so in ways that punish victims and fail to punish perpetrators appropriately.

Girls who physically fight back may be punished not only by the boys who attack them, but also by school authorities unfairly and unevenly. The narratives of girls who are harassed and who respond actively to that harassment are filled with stories of unjust punishment. One girl who was backed into a corner and physically touched by two or three boys in her classroom was punished by her teacher for running out of the room, while her harassers went unpunished (Stein, 1999, pp. 13-14). The same teachers and principals who observe multiple incidents of harassment of girls and fail to respond at all seem to quickly notice as well as discipline girls for striking back at their harassers. Girls report being caught hitting their attackers, who typically deny any provocation–and it is the girls, not the boys, whose stories are disbelieved (Stein, 1999). This dynamic appeared in a recent legal case for peer sexual harassment from Indiana: a "more physically developed" 8th grade girl, the frequent target of harassment and sexual remarks from boys in her class, jabbed one of these boys with a pen after he "threatened to poke her breast and made a lewd, offensive remark" (*B.A.L. v. Apple,* 2001). Both students were sent to the principal's office, where the boy was sent back without any punishment, while the girl was given a choice between two days suspension or three swats of a paddle. Perhaps the most egregious example of punishing and blaming the victim hails from a 1999 case from Colorado in which a school janitor found a male student who had been awarded privileges as a "janitor's assistant" raping a female student with cerebral palsy and told him to "clean up the mess" (*Murrell v. School District,* 1999). In a later meeting between the female student's mother and the school principal, the principal declined to investigate the incident or punish the attacker in any way, even though he admitted engaging in the assault. Instead, the principal responded by suspending the victim for "behavior which is detrimental to the welfare, safety or morals of other pupils or school personnel." These and other cases illustrate how school personnel can acquiesce or support the excesses of a gendered peer culture. To punish girls who engage in resistance to the sexual harassment culture of schools, whether that resistance is in the form of trying to hold their harassers accountable or in the form of physical resistance, implicates school officials in the reinforcement of the cultural dynamics that they would like to extinguish.

Finally, another common approach to dealing with sexual harassment between children in the same classroom is to move the perpetrator to another class. This reflects the approach of restraining order laws that enforce "no contact" between domestic violence offenders and their victims, and the appeal of other solutions that require the victim to leave her abusive mate. The unfortunate fact is that battered women are often attacked and killed after they leave, a phenomenon which is well known as "separation assault" (Mahoney, 1991). It has long been recognized by battered women's advocates that leaving the relationship may solve the immediate problem for the victim (if it doesn't create greater ones), but it leaves the perpetrator free to move on to a new victim–which happens in the vast majority of cases.

A similar principle applies to children involved in peer harassment. In one recent case, a 6th grade girl in Georgia was repeatedly touched during class in front of her teacher and classmates by a boy in her class before any action was taken by the school principal (*Clark v. Bibb County Board of Education*, 2001). After he was moved to another class, he continued to harass her in the hallways and other public spaces of the school. When the victim's parents asked that he be transferred to another school, their request was declined–although they did offer to transfer their daughter to another school. Perhaps even more startling is a case from Virginia involving a kindergarten boy who exhibited acts of sexual aggression towards his classmates, including "humping" them, fondling their genitals, and initiating acts of sexual intimacy. After several children and their parents complained, the boy was simply moved to another class and a folder about his behavior placed on his teacher's desk (*Doe v. Sabine Parish Board,* 1998). Not surprisingly, he began to assault his new classmates shortly after his arrival in his new classroom.

Whatever the stereotype that moves school officials to simply change the physical location of the sexual harasser and think they've solved the problem, it is likely to be ineffective. Although it is a punishment to remove a child from his familiar classroom and that action will keep the immediate victim safe during classtime, the Clark case, which is consistent with the AAUW statistics, reminds us that harassment can and often does occur in the hallways and other public spaces of a school. Failing to guard against victims' vulnerabilities outside the classroom is a mistake that may incur liability for a school under Monroe. In addition, a change of location creates new opportunities for the harasser to find new victims. Clearly, school officials may use removal of a child who is sexually harassing his classmates in their repertoire of appropriate responses, but they must also address the harassing conduct itself and take steps to insure that it is not simply recreated in a new classroom environment that, despite having different children, operates according to the basic principles of most school societies.

CONCLUSION

Peer sexual harassment occurs in a context that sometimes may be hard for school service providers to see, or before they expect to see it. Sexual harassment is aggressive behavior, not "normal flirting and teasing," although its perceived normality can be part of the problem. We have suggested that aggressive and/or gendered behavior in school is best viewed within a contextualist framework like the school society where peer groups and social status are recognized as key organizing factors. As our narrative cases suggest, even well-meaning school service providers can unintentionally collaborate with peer culture dynamics that normalize or reinforce behaviors that to the rest of us clearly suggest harassment. They can also dismiss the challenges made by girls in protest of unwanted sexual behavior. Among researchers and educators alike, attention needs to be paid to the peer groups of the victim and the harasser, their behavioral characteristics and ties to the larger peer culture. School authorities need to ask questions about who else was present (as bystander, encourager, co-harasser, co-victim, or victim protector) before, during, and after harassment, and they should assess to what degree the students involved seem to be leaders or otherwise have social status among their peers (Farmer, 2000). In particular, school service providers should not assume that the instigators of harassment (whether out in-front or behind the scenes) are rejected, unpopular children on the periphery of school social life. Even popular leaders may engage in sexually harassing behavior.

We are also suggesting that the sexual harassment experienced in school by girls contains many of the same dynamics as domestic violence between adults. Understanding that victims may respond in active, aggressive ways to such harassment or retaliate for earlier harassment should be useful to officials when deciding how to punish that aggressive behavior. The way that school officials typically respond to harassment also has parallels in domestic violence intervention. By avoiding the pitfalls and errors that have plagued police and other legal personnel in domestic violence calls, school officials will be better equipped to recognize the nature of sexual harassment between children in their schools and respond in a manner that sends the appropriate messages to both victims and perpetrators. Specifically, school officials should hesitate before assuming that girls, who may be afraid to speak out against their harassers, have initiated physical aggression against a bigger, more powerful boy, as it would be a reasonable hypothesis that her aggression might be a response to ongoing or past harassment, to that boy or to his peers. The other common mistake that school officials appear to make that bears correcting is to solve the problem of harassment by moving the perpetrator to another classroom, leaving him to freely harass his victim(s) at recess, lunch, and before and after school as well as providing him with a naïve environment in which to find new victims.

We do think that a framework that encourages school officials to think more broadly about relational and societal contexts when responding to sexual harassment will make those responses more effective. If school officials are able to significantly intervene in aggression between boys and girls in grade school, the stage for how men and women treat each other as adults may be set in a very different place than it is now.

REFERENCES

Abecassis, M., Hartup, W. W., Haselager, G. J. T., Scholte, R., & van Lieshout, C. F. M. (2002). Mutual antipathies and their significance in middle childhood and early adolescence. *Child Development, 73*, 1543-56.

Adler, P. A., & Adler, P. (1998). *Peer power: Preadolescent culture and identity.* New Brunswick, NJ: Rutgers University Press.

Allen, V. L. (1981). Self, social group, and social structure: Surmises about the study of children's friendships. In S. R. Asher & J. M. Gottman (Eds.), *The development of children's friendships* (pp. 182-203). New York: Cambridge University Press.

American Association of University Women Educational Foundation (2001). *Hostile hallways: Bullying, teasing, and sexual harassment in school.* Washington, DC: American Association of University Women.

American Association for University Women Educational Foundation. (1993). *Hostile hallways: The AAUW survey on sexual harassment in America's schools.* Washington, DC: Author.

B.A.L. v. Apple, 2001 WL 1135024 (not reported), S.D. Indiana (2001).

Benenson, J., Apostoleris, N., & Parnass, J. (1998). The organization of children's same-sex peer relations. In W. M. Bukowski & A. H. N. Cillessen (Eds.), *Sociometry then and now: Building on six decades of measuring children's experiences with the peer group* (pp. 5-23). San Francisco: Jossey-Bass.

Bernard, J. (1979). *The female world.* New York: Basic Books.

Boulton, M. J. (1999). Concurrent and longitudinal relations between children's playground behavior and social preference, victimization, and bullying. *Child Development, 70,* 944-954.

Bronfenbrenner, U. (1979). *The ecology of human development: Experiments by nature and design.* Cambridge, MA: Harvard University Press.

Bruneau v. South Kortright Central School District, 935 F. Supp. 162 (N.D.N.Y. 1996).

Bukowski, W. M., Sippola, L. K., & Newcomb, A. F. (2000). Variations in patterns of attraction to same- and other-sex peers during early adolescence. *Developmental Psychology, 36,* 147-154.

Cairns, R. B., Elder, G. H., Jr., & Costello, E. J. (Eds.). (1996). *Developmental science.* New York: Cambridge University Press.

Cairns, R. B., Xie, H., & Leung, M-C. (1998). The popularity of friendship and the neglect of social networks: Toward a new balance. In W. M. Bukowski & A. H. Cillessen (Eds.), *Sociometry then and now: Building on six decades of measuring children's experiences with the peer group* (pp. 25-53). San Francisco: Jossey-Bass.

Clark v. Bibb County Board of Education, 174 f. Supp. 2d 1369 (M.D. Ga. 2001)

Coleman, J. (1961). *The adolescent society.* Glencoe, IL: Free Press.

Craig, W. M., Pepler, D., Connolly, J., & Henderson, K. (2001). Developmental context of peer harassment in early adolescence: the role of puberty and the peer group. In J. Juvonen & S. Graham (Eds.), *Peer harassment in school: The plight of the vulnerable and victimized* (pp. 242-261). New York: Guilford.

Davis. v. Monroe County Board of Education, 526 U.S. 629 (1999).

Doe v. Sabine Parish Board, 24 F. Supp. 2d 655 (W.D. La. 1998).

Eder, D., Evans, C. C., & Parker, S. (1995). *School talk: Gender and adolescent culture.* New Brunswick, NJ: Rutgers University Press.

Estell, D. B., Farmer, T. W., Van Acker, R., Pearl, R., & Rodkin, P. C. (in press). Heterogeneity in the relationship between popularity and aggression: Individual, group, and classroom influences. In S. C. Peck (Ed.), *Use of person-centered approaches in the study of human development in context.* San Francisco: Jossey Bass.

Farmer, T. W. (2000). Social dynamics of aggressive and disruptive behavior in school: Implications for behavior consultation. *Journal of Educational and Psychological Consultation, 11,* 299-322.

Farmer, T. W., Leung, M-C., Pearl, R., Rodkin, P. C., Cadwallader, T. W., & Van Acker, R. (2002). Deviant or diverse peer groups? The peer affiliations of aggressive elementary students. *Journal of Educational Psychology, 94,* 611-620.

Fischer, K., Vidmar, N., & Ellis, R. (1993). The culture of battering and the role of mediation in domestic violence cases. *Southern Methodist University Law Review* (Special Issue on Alternative Dispute Resolution), *46,* 2117-73.

Gorman, A. H., Kim, J., & Schimmelbusch, A. (2002). The attributes adolescents associate with peer popularity and teacher preference. *Journal of School Psychology, 40,* 143-165.

Graham, S., & Juvonen, J. (2002). Ethnicity, peer harassment, and adjustment in middle school: An exploratory study. *Journal of Early Adolescence, 22,* 173-199.

Hodges, E. V. E., & Card, N. (Eds.). (in press). *The (unwanted) company they keep: Enemy relationships in childhood and adolescence.* San Francisco: Jossey Bass.

Hodges, E. V. E., Malone, M. J., & Perry, D. G. (1997). Individual risk and social risk as interacting determinants of victimization in the peer group. *Developmental Psychology, 33,* 1032-1039.

LaFontana, K. M., & Cillessen, A. H. N. (2002). Children's perceptions of popular and unpopular peers: A multi-method assessment. *Developmental Psychology, 38,* 635-647.

Lewin, K. (1943). Psychology and the process of group living. *Journal of Social Psychology, 17,* 113-131.

Lippitt, R., Polansky, N., Redl, F., & Rosen, S. (1952). The dynamics of power: A field study of social influence in groups of children. In G. E. Swanson, T. M. Newcomb, & E. L. Hartley (Eds.), *Readings in social psychology* (rev. ed., pp. 623-636). New York: Holt.

Maccoby, E. E. (1998). *The two sexes: Growing up apart, coming together.* Cambridge, MA: Harvard University Press.

Mahoney, M. R. (1991). Legal images of battered women: Redefining the issue of separation. *Michigan Law Review, 90,* 1-94.

Merten, D. E. (1997). The meaning of meanness: Popularity, competition, and conflict among junior high school girls. *Sociology of Education, 70,* 175-191.

Milgram, S. (1977). *The individual in a social world: Essays and experiments.* New York: McGraw Hill.

Murnen, S. K., & Smolak, L. (2000). The experience of sexual harassment among grade-school students: Early socialization of female subordination. *Sex Roles: A Journal of Research, 43,* 17-25.

Murrell v. School Dist. No. 1, Denver, Colo., 186 F.3d 1238 (Colo. 1999).

Nisbett, R. E., & Cohen, D. (1996). *Culture of honor: The psychology of violence in the South.* Boulder, CO: Westview Press.

O'Connell, P., Pepler, D., & Craig, W. (1999). Peer involvement in bullying: Insights and challenges for intervention. *Journal of Adolescence, 22,* 437-452.

Parker, J. G., & Seal, J. (1996). Forming, losing, renewing, and replacing friendships: Applying temporal parameters to the assessment of children's friendship experiences. *Child Development, 67,* 2248-2268.

Pellegrini, A. D., Bartini, M., & Brooks, F. (1999). School bullies, victims, and aggressive victims: Factors relating to group affiliation and victimization in early adolescence. *Journal of Educational Psychology, 91,* 216-224.

Phillips, L. (1998). *The girls report and what we need to know about growing up female.* New York: National Council for Research on Women.

Prinstein, M. J., & Cillessen, A. H. N. (2003). Forms and functions of adolescent peer aggression associated with high levels of peer status. *Merrill Palmer Quarterly, 49,* 310-342.

Rodkin, P. C. (2002). *I think you're cool: Social status and group support for aggressive boys and girls.* Invited address to the 8th Triannual Meeting of the Northeast Social Development Consortium, New York.

Rodkin, P. C., Farmer, T. W., Pearl, R., & Van Acker, R. (2000). Heterogeneity of popular boys: Antisocial and prosocial configurations. *Developmental Psychology, 36,* 14-24.

Rodkin, P. C., Pearl, R., Farmer, T. W., & Van Acker, R. (in press). Enemies in the gendered societies of middle childhood: Prevalence, stability, associations with social status and aggression. In E. V. E. Hodges & N. Card (Eds.), *The (unwanted) company they keep: Enemy relationships in childhood and adolescence.* San Francisco: Jossey Bass.

Romano, P. (2001). *Davis v. Monroe County Board of Education:* Title IX recipients' 'head in the sand' approach to peer sexual harassment may incur liability. *Journal of Law and Education, 30,* 63-84.

Ross, L., & Nisbett, R. E. (1991). *The person and the situation: Perspectives of social psychology.* New York: McGraw Hill.

Salmivalli, C., Huttunen, A., & Lagerspetz, K. M. J. (1997). Peer networks and bullying in schools. *Scandinavian Journal of Psychology, 38,* 305-312.

Sherif, M. (1956). Experiments in group conflict. *Scientific American, 195,* 54-58.

Stein, N. (1999). *Classrooms and courtrooms: Facing sexual harassment in K-12 schools.* New York: Teachers College Press.

Sutton, J., Smith, P. K., & Swettenham, J. (1999). Bullying and 'theory of mind': A critique of the 'social skills deficit' view of anti-social behaviour. *Social Development, 8,* 117-127.

Thorne, B. (1993). *Gender play: Girls and boys in school.* New Brunswick, NJ: Rutgers University Press.

Underwood, M. K., Schockner, A. E., & Hurley, J. C. (2001). Children's responses to same- and other-gender peers: An experimental investigation with 8-, 10-, and 12-year-olds. *Developmental Psychology, 37,* 362-372.

Index

Abusive Behavior Inventory, 86,90
Academic performance
  of bullies, 158-159,164
  of victims, 27,28,123,126,129-130
    gender differences in, 34
Academic self-efficacy, of victims,
    33-34,38
Aggression
  by bullies, 163-164,165,166,167
    as basis for peer rejection, 160
    as basis for popularity, 160
    gender differences in, 166,169
  male
    cultural values related to, 186
    in kindergarten students, 191
    social status factors in, 184-186
    women's attraction to, 186
  socially manipulative, by girls,
    102
  by victims, 28,35,141,149,150,
    152-153
Alcohol abuse, by victims, 140
American Association of University
    Women, sexual harassment
    surveys by, 12,13,82-83,86,90,
    94,178,179,181-182,191-192
Anger, in dating violence victims,
    82-83
Anxiety
  in dating violence victims, 82-83
  gender differences in, 34
  in victims, 35,36,37-38,40,48,126,
    127,145-147,151,152,153
    cluster analysis of, 91,93
    gender differences in, 39
Athleticism, of bullies, 163-164,166,
    167,169,171-172

Attitudes, toard bullying, 63-79
  of bullies, 66,71,73,74-75
  of victims, 71,73,75
Austria, immigrant children's
    interethnic relationships in,
    99-116
  children from former Yugoslavia,
    106-107,108-109,110,111,112
  Turkish/Kurdish children, 106,107,
    108-109,110,112

Beck Depression Inventory, 32
Borderwork, 183-184
*Bruneau v. South Kortright Central
    School District,* 189,190
Bullies
  academic performance of,
    158-159, 164
  aggression by,
    163-164,165,166,167
    as basis for peer rejection, 160
    as basis for popularity, 160
    gender differences in, 166,169
  athleticism of,
    163-164,166,167,169, 171-172
  characteristics of, 158-159
  cliques of, 185-186
  delinquency of, 65,158-159
  depression in, 65,158-159,167,168
  female, 4,166,169
  leadership ability of,
    164,165,167,168,169
  loneliness in, 65,158-159,167,168
  motivation for bullying, 74-75
  peer rejection of, 159-160

SPECIAL 25%-OFF DISCOUNT!

Order a copy of this book with this form or online at:
http://www.haworthpress.com/store/product.asp?sku=4982
Use Sale Code BOF25 in the online bookshop to receive 25% off!

Bullying, Peer Harassment, and Victimization in the Schools
The Next Generation of Prevention

____ in softbound at $18.71 (regularly $24.95) (ISBN: 0-7890-2229-X)
____ in hardbound at $29.96 (regularly $39.95) (ISBN: 0-7890-2228-1)

COST OF BOOKS _____

Outside USA/ Canada/
Mexico: Add 20% _____

POSTAGE & HANDLING _____
(US: $4.00 for first book & $1.50
for each additional book)
Outside US: $5.00 for first book
& $2.00 for each additional book)

SUBTOTAL _____

in Canada: add 7% GST _____

STATE TAX _____
(CA, MIN, NY, OH, & SD residents please
add appropriate local sales tax

FINAL TOTAL _____
(if paying in Canadian funds, convert
using the current exchange rate,
UNESCO coupons welcome)

❑ **BILL ME LATER:** ($5 service charge will be added)
(Bill-me option is good on US/Canada/
Mexico orders only; not good to jobbers,
wholesalers, or subscription agencies.)

❑ **Signature** _____

❑ **Payment Enclosed: $** _____

❑ **PLEASE CHARGE TO MY CREDIT CARD:**

❑ Visa ❑ MasterCard ❑ AmEx ❑ Discover
❑ Diner's Club ❑ Eurocard ❑ JCB

Account #_____

Exp Date _____

Signature_____
*(Prices in US dollars and subject to
change without notice.)*

PLEASE PRINT ALL INFORMATION OR ATTACH YOUR BUSINESS CARD		
Name		
Address		
City	State/Province	Zip/Postal Code
Country		
Tel	Fax	
E-Mail		

May we use your e-mail address for confirmations and other types of information? ❑Yes❑ No
We appreciate receiving your e-mail address. Haworth would like to e-mail special discount
offers to you, as a preferred customer. **We will never share, rent, or exchange your e-mail
address.** We regard such actions as an invasion of your privacy.

Order From Your Local Bookstore or Directly From
The Haworth Press, Inc.
10 Alice Street, Binghamton, New York 13904-1580 • USA
Call Our toll-free number (1-800-429-6784) / Outside US/Canada: (607) 722-5857
Fax: 1-800-895-0582 / Outside US/Canada: (607) 771-0012
E-Mail your order to us: Orders@haworthpress.com

Please Photocopy this form for your personal use.
www.HaworthPress.com

BOF03